YOGA FOR HANDICAPPED PEOPLE

Barbara Brosnan

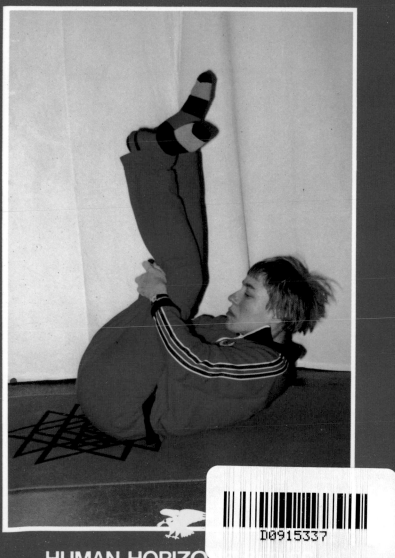

HUMAN HORIZONS SERIES

YOGA FOR HANDICAPPED PEOPLE

HUMAN HORIZONS SERIES

YOGA FOR HANDICAPPED PEOPLE

Barbara Brosnan, M.B., Ch.B.

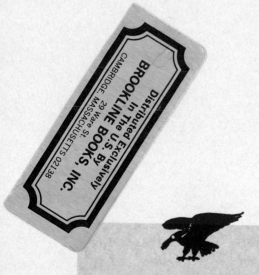

Distributed In The U.S. Exclusively By
BROOKLINE BOOKS, INC.
CAMBRIDGE, 29 Ware St.
MASSACHUSETTS 02138

A CONDOR BOOK
SOUVENIR PRESS (E&A) LTD

First published 1982 by Souvenir Press
(Educational & Academic) Ltd,
43 Great Russell Street, London WC1B 3PA
and simultaneously in Canada

ISBN 0 285 64947 7 casebound
ISBN 0 285 64952 3 paperback

Printed in Great Britain by
Ebenezer Baylis & Son Ltd,
The Trinity Press, Worcester, and London

Contents

Acknowledgements

First and foremost I am indebted to my employers Servite Houses Ltd, who gave me time off to write this book. After them I have a great number of people to thank — Mary Dargie for many hours spent on the line drawings for the postures; Wendy and Yvonne for deciphering some very bad handwriting and putting no fewer than four drafts into type-script; Mary S. and Sylvia for spending whole days together checking and working on the postures by following text and line drawings. Mary S. wielded a corrective pencil too, tightening the style and generally making the meaning clear.

Furthermore I have to thank Ann and Massiah for patiently posing in the correct or modified postures for the photographer, and of course, the number one yoga-squad at Servite House — Derek, Trevor, Gloria, Jenny and Sylvia, whose faces laugh up at you from their attempted modified postures. They worked hard and long to reach the standard photographed, as did the chair group, comprising Jean, Leslie and Peg. Indeed without all of these the book would not have come into being.

Speaking personally I am deeply grateful to my father who many years ago taught me the importance of breath control in my own life, and to Malcolm Strutt, to whose classes I went — and who advised on the starting of our classes here in Servite House. Lastly I must mention Howard Kent whose enthusiasm in the cause of yoga as therapy — in particular for M. S. sufferers — has always been an inspiration, and whose Yoga for Health Foundation at Ickwell Bury is not only a peaceful haven to which I happily retreat, but also a splendid place for refuelling, and learning.

The author would also like to thank Joe Appel for photograph No. 4, and John Bignall for the rest of the photographs.

Author's Note

It is taken for granted that yoga teachers will make sure that their pupils have contacted their own doctors before coming to start yoga classes, and that their doctors approve. All DIY enthusiasts, relatives and friends should also make sure that their doctor is in the picture, and that they are not embarking on anything that could in any way be harmful.

How to use this Book

It is probably not a good idea to read this book straight through, but to keep it on hand for reference after reading the most useful chapters.

The teacher who finds herself approached by handicapped people who want to learn yoga will find Chapters Two, Three, Eight and Nine of most value. The simple posture content of Chapters Five, Six and Seven, the easy breath control exercises of Chapter Four will be very familiar to her already. Chapter Ten may contain an unfamiliar meditation or two—it is always handy to come across some fresh ones—and Chapter One may clarify her mind as to the very great value of yoga for a handicapped person.

For a handicapped person himself, his relatives and friends, it is a good idea to read Chapter One, then turn to Chapter Three, study it and try out the warming up and breathing routines before moving to Chapter Five. A check with Chapter Eight—for the specific disability or the section on the elderly—and you are in business! Once 'hooked', Chapter Four should be studied carefully, and some of the breathing procedures practised before proceeding to Chapters Six and Seven. You and your helpers are now yoga practitioners—carry on, but look for a teacher too. Refer to Glossary number two, when you come across an anatomical or physiological word that is strange, but it is better not to get bogged down with Appendix I till later on. Some books from the Bibliography, the simple ones, could be useful early, so get them and read them in conjunction with this one.

Happy practising!

Foreword

This book sets out to show that the practice of yoga, not just the postures but the whole yogic way of life, has a great deal to offer a person with a handicap.

It is not meant to be a general text book of yoga — there are plenty of these available, written at all levels from the very simple to the highly scientific or abstruse. It is however written with a dual readership in mind.

It is for yoga teachers who would like to integrate people with a handicap into their classes, or to run classes especially for them, and would like guidance on the matter. This I have set out to provide, although I believe that a good yoga teacher will know intuitively what to try, how to help, what to avoid, and how far to go. It is also meant for any handicapped persons — and/or their parents and relatives — who might feel disposed to try it out, on their own, in order to discover what there is in yoga for them. Once they are convinced of its value — as I feel sure they will be — then they can look around for a teacher. Some thirty years' experience has confirmed me in the belief that it is not possible to try out yoga without wanting both to go further and to know more.

For the second group the text has purposely been kept simple, and the diagrams made as explicit as possible. Go on — try it — you cannot possibly come to any harm, you can come to much good — and you'll get a lot of fun in the process! Whether you want to make yoga a way of life, or just to dabble to see if 'there really is anything in it for me' or 'if it could help So-and-so at all', there is scope for everybody.

To those readers who ask why there is nothing in the book about diet, when it plays such an important part in physical health and mental and emotional stability — that is the reason. It is so important that even a whole chapter could no more than touch the fringe of the subject.

Suffice it to say that the yoga practitioner gradually finds him- or herself turning away from meat, inclining more and more to simple grains, nuts, fruits and vegetables. Alcohol and tobacco lose their meaning.

There is no need to force this, as a real awareness of your self develops, along with breath control, calmness and freedom from tension, so the taste for simple whole foods, pure and unadulterated, stemming from life not death, will grow. Don't become a crank and a bore, but nevertheless — let it happen to you.

Note In order to simplify the writing and make the instructions clearer, the teacher is always spoken of as 'she' throughout, and the pupil as 'he'. The helper is also a 'she'. No sex discrimination is intended!

1: Therapeutic Potential of Yoga

The practice of yoga colours and enhances the whole of life: the practitioner gets out of it in proportion to what he puts into it, only a hundredfold. The field of yoga extends from the practice of simple physical exercises, to the development of advanced mental and spiritual powers. It is much more than — to quote one or two common definitions —

1) a technique whereby you learn to relax;
2) balanced exercises promoting physical well-being;
3) a means towards peace of mind in the midst of stress and tension; or
4) a guide to self-realisation.

One of the greatest of today's problems is dis-harmony within the person — dis-harmony, dis-ease. The coordination of slow, thoughtful movements with slow, thoughtful breathing as found in yoga creates harmony throughout the whole individual. Breath, movement of body, and the power of the mind are directed towards one goal, resulting in integration within the individual: 'a union of body, mind and spirit', which is another one of the definitions of yoga. The dis-harmony becomes harmonised.

As we grow older we all recognise that our body is becoming lazy and stiff; it is somehow less responsive. Some of us are also aware that our mind is even more so! The uniqueness of yoga lies in the fact that as the body relaxes, opening up and acquiring a fluidity of movement, so does the mind. Together with this, there comes the releasing of emotion: with that, tension drains quietly away.

Herein lies the therapeutic potential of yoga: the production of increasing interior calmness, and freedom from tension. This calmness is not 'apathy': 'awareness' and the ability to concentrate the mind are both increased. The yoga practitioner will speak with joy of feeling himself coming steadily more and more alive; of his whole person feeling amalgamated into one harmonious whole. As the result of patient and persevering practice of yoga, energy is generated and can be stored; it can then be brought into use precisely as and when needed.

One fundamental concomitant of working on yoga postures is the acquisition of the ability to relax—an ability which comes naturally to animals. We see it every day in the comfortable, enviable sprawl of dogs and cats, or the sudden totally relaxed collapse of a small child between one step and the next. But after childhood this is an art that has to be relearned, and the yoga postures teach it, so minimising the actual physiological effects of stress. Ten minutes of really deep relaxation is the equivalent of seven hours sleep. Regular relaxation results in inner peace and harmony, deep awareness—mental and physical—and emotional control allied to coordination of movement: in fact a state of absolute health.

The benefits accruing from the regular, intelligent and careful practice of yoga follow whatever the age of the individual, however late in life the start, and—to a greater or lesser degree—whatever the physical state in which they start. Moreover they are lifelong benefits.

At all times, in fact, the body's ability to adapt or to develop anew is phenomenal. If some physical effort is made, working carefully with the breath, even minimal movements can stimulate the viscera and improve their functioning, stimulate the endocrine system so that the functioning of every ductless gland improves, and so stimulate the muscles of the spine that the whole body comes in line. Movement and breath, working together, improve the circulation, and this in turn affects the nervous systems (central and autonomic). Thus a state of general physical well-being is brought about. Moreover the calmness, freedom from emotional imbalance and release of tension already described, have a tranquillising effect on the person as a whole.

These benefits of yoga as a way of life for everybody are equally true as far as physically or mentally handicapped people are concerned; but over and beyond all of them, there are some particular advantages which apply in their case.

Disability, as dealt with here, comprises

a) physical disability, whether congenital (that is, present from birth), or acquired at some point during life; whether it be stationary (that is once acquired, it remains a disability of that same degree) or progressive (meaning that it gets steadily worse);

b) mental handicap—of all levels, from very low functioning to just below 'normal', and with or without accompanying physical handicap.

It must be admitted that at the present time, in spite of the welfare state, the odds are still stacked against handicapped people. Their education (difficult anyway in view of the disability, the need for various treatments, time away from school for operations perhaps, the presence of communication defects and so forth) is for instance frequently sub-standard, largely due to lack of facilities. The cause for this may be purely financial, but sometimes it can be due to plain lack of vision on the part of local authorities. Their recreational needs are also inadequately met, and for the same reasons.

Then there are difficulties that arise from disabled people themselves, not inherent in the disability, but inherent in having a disability. Frequently they are subject to self-doubt, they lack confidence, and have a poor self-image—these factors result from their previous lack of success in all directions, as well as from their awareness of their own abnormality. These attitudes on their part are further triggered off by our attitudes. Many people want to sweep handicapped people under the carpet, pretend that they don't exist, even think maybe (and unfortunately *show* the thought) that they *ought not* to exist! Or worse still, they want to organise them, run their lives—at the very least make all decisions for them. So often the tendency is to over-protect a handicapped person by doing everything for him, thinking this is a kindness. No wonder they, handicapped people, develop such a poor self-image, such deep-rooted feelings of inferiority. Add to this the difficulty in concentration, so often a striking feature of both physical and mental disability, the lack of energy that sometimes accompanies both, and it is easy to see why tension plays such a large part in a handicapped life. In fact, two of the most important factors affecting the life and happiness of a handicapped person are

1) his high degree of tension;
2) his repeated lack of success, if not his outright failure, in all spheres.

These factors are often present in someone who appears on the surface to be most balanced and integrated.

Let us now consider the value of the practice of yoga for such a one. It is a daily occupation (*should* be practised daily) wherein each individual works at his own pace — a pace which is meant to be slow and unstrained. It is entirely non-competitive — it couldn't matter less 'how far' the other people in the group are getting in a given posture — yet it can be done alongside other people, with all the fun of 'sharing' classes, the companionship. It requires no special equipment, (though it is a good thing for each to have his own yoga mat), so there need be no initial expense. Once embarked upon, it is a lifelong activity — there is no need to give it up at 50, 60, 70, 80, or 90; nor is it necessary to start early — it is possible to begin at any age. *And* the pupil sees noticeable results quickly. In short, he *succeeds*. Not according to book standards, perhaps, but progress is evident, right from the beginning. He can *feel* this, and *watch* it grow! A spell 'off practice' for any reason whatever does not matter much: there is some stiffness on starting again, some piece of acquired flexibility goes, no more, and it soon comes back again.

The practice of yoga teaches body posture, and encourages the right posture — in time it can overcome such deformities as have crept in with the years, even if these are quite severe. As we have already seen, it teaches relaxation, combatting the ever present tension. What is more, it leaves the individual armed with a method for overcoming his own tension whenever it seems about to seize hold. An understanding of both its causes and effects develops — so that the yoga practitioner becomes his own therapist! It greatly helps concentration, by combining physical effort with 'one-pointedness' in the mind. As a result the depressing feeling of inferiority gradually but steadily diminishes and self-confidence is built up instead.

The actual physical movements achieved — with or without help — improve the overall circulation and strengthen the heart. Consequently, oxygenation is increased throughout the body, and with improved oxygenation comes improvement in the whole level of functioning. And the handicapped person discovers a means of storing up energy within himself, so that it is always to hand, and can be called upon at will.

Every posture can be simultaneously conceived of as a) the perfect posture as seen in text-book illustrations, b) the near-perfect posture as demonstrated in the class, and c) the 'thought into and through' posture of the handicapped person. While achieving what of each posture he can, maybe with help, maybe entirely on his own, the handicapped person learns how to function within a disability, how to help himself in spite of the disability, how to compensate for a given restriction by doing something else.

He may even learn how to overcome a specific disability. Some of the skills learned are of protective value against the hazards routine to handicapped people. For instance he may learn to get up, at any rate as far as a sitting position, after he has fallen flat on the floor. It is surprising how many 'fit' people with cerebral palsy cannot achieve this: they may have absolutely no idea of the supportive and pushing rôle of the arm! Continued practice may produce definite physical improvement, or avert increasing disability. This is particularly true in the spine. The often uncoordinated movement of the mentally handicapped person, or the poor movement of the physically handicapped person, allows the spine to stiffen up and lose all its mobility, thus producing much pain, still further limitation of movement, and hence further lack of coordination.

The practice of yoga produces a sensation of feeling good, feeling well, and on top of our form, so it quickly provides its own motivation for continuing, for working away at the postures. There is rapid development of the awareness of self-mastery, a progress in self-discipline with its accompanying feeling of independence, a knowledge of being a person in one's own right.

Yoga provides 'success' for the handicapped person. He is doing something that normal people do. Consequently it can to a remarkable extent, modify, improve his whole attitude to his disability. Away goes the chip on the shoulder; his frustration lessens; annoyance and irritability come under the control of relaxation, the appearance of apathy characteristic of some disabled people vanishes. The limp acceptance, acquiescence of inertia, gives way to a genuine acceptance of being a person with a disability, of living with it and getting on with the job of living, in spite of it. On the other hand the occasional obstinate insistence on 'independence', that refusal to accept any help, which can make life so much more difficult both for the handicapped person himself and for other people, all that disappears too. An integrated person simply and naturally accepts the help he needs, as and when he needs it.

Yoga can be practised in a chair, or in a wheelchair, on the floor, or while lying in bed. It does not have to include sitting or standing. Unless actually ill, anyone who can do it in bed can do it on the floor—though it may take a little time to convince him of this! Postures can be modified to suit the individual degree of physical handicap, no matter how severe; they can be simplified for the mentally handicapped, made 'fun' and a joy for the emotionally imbalanced whose energy yoga channels productively. The overall calming effect is clearly seen in the relaxation period at the end of a class, when all, no matter what their problems, lie in utter peace and tranquillity; tension, anxious breathing, jerks, fidgets, all are stilled. There is deep personal satisfaction in this.

For a physically handicapped person, slight movements are of great value— no matter how minimal they may be. The means are really every bit as valuable as the end. Moreover, each posture is of value, no matter how much of it has to be *done for* the person, however small the effort possible on his own. For example, the increased flow of blood to the head and the stimulation of the thyroid resulting from the shoulder stand is equally present, whether the person has done it on his own, or, as is often necessary for a spastic person, he has been helped up into the posture and then been literally held there. And the gentle squeezing, massaging of the gut that takes place when anyone relaxes into the pose of a child is similarly produced when that person, seated in a wheelchair, is helped forward and down into the rag-doll position, and is then just held there, with arms and head totally relaxed, chest on knees.

2: Hints to Teachers and Others

The Class
Ordinary yoga classes usually involve fairly large numbers of students—anything from twelve to twenty. With handicapped people, a number of considerations may modify this.

Even with a moderate degree of physical handicap, some help is necessary with most postures—if this were not the case the individual would be able to attend an ordinary class. Consequently the number of pupils in the class at any one time will depend upon the number of helpers available, their experience, and the number of helpers the teacher feels she can oversee at one time. Help is often needed on a one-to-one basis, and sometimes the handicapped person may need two people helping him in order to attempt the postures at all. This reduces the number of pupils it is possible to have in any one class. The teacher herself may be able to cope with two slightly handicapped people, and give them sufficient help at the same time as overseeing the whole class. In that case, with two or three helpers, a class of five or six, but not more, is a possibility.

Although yoga is non-competitive, there is both simulation and 'fun' in a group working at it together. To have two people of rather similar disability together often proves a great incentive to progress for both. There is also an advantage in having one or two people without any very definite physical handicap in the class—elderly people, perhaps.

Where physical disability is extreme, and particularly in the early stages when there is everything to learn, it is best to have one pupil with the teacher, plus one or even two helpers.

When considering mentally handicapped people for yoga sessions, decisions will first depend on whether or not the pupil has an additional physical handicap. Where there is no physical handicap, and the mental handicap is minimal, the pupil should be integrated into an ordinary yoga class. Pupils with no physical handicap but relatively severe or very severe mental handicap are best together in a class on their own—they are too energetic to be combined with physically handicapped pupils, and require a different teaching approach from those who are not mentally handicapped (see page 27). If, however, the predominant factor is the physical handicap, then, regardless of the mental handicap, such a person should be with other physically handicapped people—unless it so happens that there are three or four people of similar heavy dual handicap, meriting a class to themselves.

The Teacher

The first essential for the teacher is belief: she must believe strongly in what she is doing, must be convinced that she is broadening the horizon, enlarging the life style of her pupils, that in imparting a skill she is offering an art that will greatly benefit her pupil as a whole, helping him physically, mentally and emotionally. Hence it is clear that the greater the teacher's knowledge of yoga, her personal experience of it and faith in it, the better. As for any teacher, it is her job to arouse and sustain interest, and to bring gaiety and joy to the class. The better an actual practical teacher she is, then the happier for all concerned! (Good teachers are born, we know, but the techniques can be acquired, and are well worth acquiring.)

The second essential for any teacher of yoga to handicapped people must be complete confidence with regard to the handicap. Nursing knowledge or other experience with handicapped people, though not essential, can be of value here. Increasingly, qualified yoga teachers are becoming involved with handicapped people, learning about them and then teaching them. (Ignorance can be terrifying both to teacher and pupil, and it often leads to too little being demanded of the pupil because the teacher does not feel safe!) Medical knowledge can also be useful, but is not in the least necessary.

In short, an *observant* person, who will take the trouble to learn about disability, and who enjoys doing yoga herself, believing in it completely, will make an excellent teacher for handicapped people.

There is nothing against a DIY approach either, and a parent or relative willing to follow a yoga book and try it out on themselves, and then on their handicapped relative, *can* do really well. To start with, the relative has one great advantage—that of not being afraid of the disability! She is used to coping with it through all the day-to-day problems of living at home. She should not be put off from trying yoga by the idea that it is all too difficult and complicated—it can be very very simple. In all probability she will quickly find that she wants to know more and more, both for herself *and* for the handicapped relative, and so set about learning at established classes.

Approach to the Class
The teacher may demonstrate the completed 'perfect' pose. But for the physically handicapped pupil, a demonstration is not always of much value—it may entail too much of what he cannot do, and so discourage him. However he can be told to 'think through' to the perfect posture—'imagine and feel' it, even though he can't get there. Some do this, others prefer to think just a little 'further on' than they can reach. Simple explanations in words, however, are always necessary: keep the knees straight, straighten up your back, stretch the arms as straight as you can up over the head. Thus the pupil can understand the reason for the physical prompt he is being given—the hand lifting the arm under the elbow, the knee in the back as a support to straighten it, the hands pulling his shoulders back. On occasions though, the pupil should not be helped but left to do just what he can of the posture, entirely on his own, no matter how infinitesimal.

Physically handicapped people are usually very realistic and basic in their approach. They have come to yoga to get something out of it, and, in the initial stages at least, the physical side of things will loom much larger in their minds than any idea of wholeness and personal integration, or any desire to develop inner awareness. As yet they may not recognise their own degree of tension, or their own emotional imbalance. To start with, the teacher must appeal to them on this essentially basic level. Intensity, and anything that will appear to the class as high flown 'jargon', must be avoided. In the early stages at least, a simple matter-of-fact approach is what the teacher should aim for. Her own enthusiasm will shine through, her fundamental belief in the value of what she is doing—and this will have its effect. Encouragement of the pupil should be lavish. And there is nothing as encouraging to the teacher as to see the pupil's rapid improvement in mobility, and agility. Awkward and ungainly though this mobility and agility may be, it will soon be seen to exist where it never existed before!

Where the handicapped people in the class are children, the teacher has to bring in an element of fun, of game playing all the time. There should be more movement—as far as this is possible—and less holding in the poses; it is vitally important not to overtax youthful stamina, which is far short of the adult's. Too much concentration should not be demanded. Time given over to breathing exercises should be relatively short, and the time of relaxation/meditation without direction—that is the silent period at the end—should be short. It should be brought to an end *before* any child starts fidgeting.

Intelligent but very physically handicapped children, even at a young age—seven or thereabouts—will like to imitate, and can be helped to imitate when put on the floor. The younger the better for this, provided there is no long holding or being held in a posture; for the slow gentle movements, the bending and stretching, are among the best forms of physiotherapy. Later the intelligent youngster will like to see the pictures, and have the functioning of his own body explained to him—also the value of the various postures. Simple breathing exercises should be taught, but without retention. A good teacher will instinctively make use of the child's imagination, particularly in developing respiratory control, by talking of blowing candles out, spouting water. The teacher has accomplished much in relation to inspiration if she succeeds in lengthening exhalation.

Music forms a most valuable adjunct to the end relaxation period, and chanting to the warming up session, as well as to any final period of relaxation-cum-meditation.

A short meditation with a real candle flame, or listening to the ticking of a loud clock, proves popular, and children will love to bring their own abstract mandalas from the art class to their yoga sessions.

The value of starting yoga really young is that the stiffness that so often comes round about puberty can be avoided. This is where the DIY at home approach can be invaluable. The development of increased mobility and coordination in the young pupil is often even more rapid and noticeable than in the elderly one.

The Helpers

As already mentioned, one-to-one is normally ideal, but two helpers to one physically handicapped person may sometimes be necessary; and one helper to two or even three pupils is a possibility where the handicap is minimal. The helpers *need* have no skill and no experience—they can acquire this quite quickly. All that is necessary is for the teacher to direct them simply and clearly: 'Put your knee behind her back so that she can straighten up; Lift the left elbow by putting your hand underneath it; Help the right arm to stretch forward, holding it at the wrist; Lift the left leg over the right just below the knee; Lift the leg well in the air, holding it just above the ankle, then let its own weight take it downwards towards the floor.'

Frequently the actual help required may need to be demonstrated, particularly if the helpers are nervous or timid and not sure how far it is safe to go. One very useful principle is to ask the pupil to give all his attention to his breathing—as it were, detach himself from the physical side of the proceedings. This brings about relaxation and enables the helper to move limbs much more freely, as they are void of tension—or at any rate nearly so.

A helper needs to be reasonably quick, able to listen, and to do just what is asked and no more. The helper to lose as quickly as possible is the one who tries to go further than the teacher, or faster, or who talks incessantly to the pupil she is helping! Only one person can talk in a class that is really working, and that is the teacher. (This is not to say that a muttered word or two or encouragement from the helper here and there is out of place.)

It is by her manner that the teacher lets a helper know how much she is valued, and how essential is the part she plays in the class. Often the helper too gets 'bitten' with the yoga bug, and will set to learning for herself. This is of great value, because her knowledge will rapidly increase, giving her an understanding of what each exercise actually involves and its purpose. At the same time her respect for those she helps will increase because now she will know exactly how difficult it is to achieve a posture well, when attempting it as a fit person — let alone as a handicapped one!

Practical aids
Some handicapped people cannot even lie on the floor without one or more cushions — under the head; under both head and shoulders; in the small of the back; or under the knees. These should be used freely. Discomfort distracts attention, so concentration is lost and effort dwindles. Simply raising the feet and legs on a low stool may be useful. Slings can be used for paralysed limbs if there is not a human hand to do the work of the sling.

Whole yoga sequences can also be carried out with the pupil sitting in an ordinary chair — a backless stool is better, though it may not be feasible. And much can be done even if the person has to remain in a wheelchair. A great deal is possible still without the person even getting out of bed — though this should be avoided, as the surface is rarely firm enough. A board under the mattress helps.

Rest
Yoga is unhurried, calm and slow, but nevertheless all sessions should include resting periods. This is particularly necessary for physically handicapped people, whose hearts are unaccustomed to running or other fast movements that increase the rate of the heart beat. Their out-of-training heart muscles cannot take too much exercise at once. The older the person the less he should be allowed to get out of breath. (See the section on the elderly at the end of Chapter Eight.)

Space and Air
It is necessary to have enough space — on the floor, there should be at least two bodies' widths between the mats, and chairs should have ample room for a helper on either side. An actual floor covering is not necessary provided each pupil

has a yoga mat or rug of some description. It is important that the room should be airy—but warm. Most people with a physical handicap feel the cold acutely and may be very sensitive to draughts. If they are living in institutions they are used to central heating, usually kept higher than in the normal household because of their poor circulation.

Clothes

The proper garb for yoga for a non-handicapped person is a leotard for a woman, shorts for a man. Physically handicapped men may find shorts too chilly, and they can be embarrassing if the pupil is wearing a urinary appliance or urostomy bag. For women a leotard, though a great joy to have, may be too chilly too, and anyway it proves a nuisance when you need to go to the loo. Slacks and a loose top are the easiest and most convenient for both men and women; bit by bit cardigans should be peeled away. But almost uniformly poor circulations should always be borne in mind—particularly on reaching the relaxation period of complete stillness at the end of the class.

Privacy

Yoga, even though the classes are fun, is a serious pursuit and spectators should not be encouraged, as they distract, and concentration really matters. The ability to concentrate is one of the more important aims. Whatever the reason, a handicapped person usually has greater difficulty with concentration than a non-handicapped person. Consequently everything possible should be done in the yoga class to improve this. Subdued lighting is beneficial—it helps each pupil to focus his attention solely on himself.

Practice

The more practice is done, the more benefit is obtained from yoga. Obviously daily practice is the best, but for people who need someone to help them all the time this is usually not possible. (Hence the need for frequent lessons.) However some part of what is done in class can be done alone. All that is necessary for this, for someone who usually works on the floor, is to put the handicapped person on a rug on the floor, and leave him to it! People working in chairs are in their chairs all the time so they can practise at any opportunity. The same is true of people in bed. Working on their own is of very real value, no matter how little the achievement, particularly if there is full attention and concentration. But a great deal of encouragement will be necessary, as this concept is alien to a physically handicapped person, used as he is to a physiotherapist working with him. (A severely mentally handicapped or emotionally imbalanced person is unlikely to practise alone at all.)

It might be possible to get a helper to work with the pupil at regular practice sessions. It is good for this to be someone who has worked with them in class, and who can therefore be relied upon to follow pattern and principle through. A member of the family who has accompanied the handicapped person to class, or who is already attempting yoga with him at home on her own, is ideal for regular practice sessions. In fact, for home workers the yoga session can be built around the day's routine for the handicapped member of the family. Even short periods of practice are of value — as little as fifteen minutes daily would soon bring incredible results. For practice there is no need for any special place: wherever the rug can be put down, or there is space for a helper round the chair will do, provided there is sufficient privacy to enable the pupil to concentrate.

Like the classes (see Chapter Three), practice should not be done when the person is too tired or has a heavy cold. Some people say not to practise when menstruating — this is not correct, yoga can greatly help premenstrual tension and the pain of both congestive and spasmodic dysmenorrhoea. Certain postures only are better not attempted (see Chapter Three). Where the first day of a period is exceptionally heavy, a few warming up exercises coupled with breathing exercises and relaxation are all that should be attempted.

Where skilled help during practice times is not available, it is better to practise *without* such help than not to practise at all. In yoga, where the mental attitude, the focussing of thought and the development of concentration are more important than what can actually be achieved by way of physical posture, such practice is bound to be valuable.

Persevering practice strengthens all the benefits that come from an ordinary yoga class, accelerates progress over all, intensifies the feeling of well-being which yoga produces, and maintains interest at a high level.

Duration of Class

Long sessions are not advisable, particularly at the beginning. The teacher is dealing with comparatively unfit people, whose hearts and lungs have little exercise tolerance. This needs to be built up. Often a mentally retarded youngster—or adult—is easily bored, as can be the emotionally imbalanced person. It is better to end the class at a point where the students would like it to go on longer—that way they come back with enthusiasm and interest. Thirty minutes rising to forty-five is best. For the comparatively fit—people with a specific disability but without the disability of being generally below par as well, such as a person with spina bifida, or some with cerebral palsy, progress can be made eventually to an hour.

In a forty-five-minute session, there should be five minutes of recollection and breathing, five minutes' warming up, twenty-five minutes of postures, and ten minutes for further breathing and final relaxation, including imagination, and concentration practice as a preparation for proper meditation work later on. In a thirty-minute session, postures should take only twenty minutes of the time, and the rest be cut down proportionately. No section must ever be omitted.

The Body as Instrument

The pupil must be given the idea that he brings an instrument to the yoga class, with which he is going to work—this is his body, and it does not matter how handicapped this body is, how little he can make it move or control its movements. Next he has to learn that his mind is to work on his body, through his body—that the mind in fact will 'finish' the posture, think it right through, even though the body may achieve little. Understanding of the way the control of the breath links with all this comes slowly. The first essential is the idea of body control and the development of the mind working positively on the body.

Place of Books, Diagrams

There are thousands of books on yoga, covering its every aspect in great detail. Some are simple, some highly abstruse.

The physically handicapped person who enjoys reading will benefit from reading them — particularly where the degree of physical handicap is great, such a one needs to understand the underlying philosophy, comprehend the value of minimal movement combined with breath control, and see the value of the posture that takes the help of other people to bring it about. Many handicapped people will not be readers, but they too will assuredly benefit from photographs of the postures completed, or partially achieved, and from line drawings. The photographs will make it all seem real, and the drawings will clarify verbal descriptions and thus reduce the number of words necessary! Full-page colour reproductions from magazines are a stimulus to a class, even though the pupils will never reach such a degree of proficiency.

Chanting, Mantras

The idea of chanting probably seems strange to everybody, not only to the handicapped, until they try it. Interestingly enough, mentally handicapped pupils in a class often bring much less self-consciousness to chanting than their more normal brethren, and hence find great release and enjoyment in it.

The use of mantras too helps concentration, 'one-pointedness of mind', and can be introduced as soon as there has been a little teaching on the preliminaries of meditation. The actual word 'meditation' need not be used for a long time — it can sound daunting to new students, and make them defensive. Early approaches to meditation however are part of the final relaxation of a class. They can be done there as a matter of course, and prepare the pupil for full meditation work later on, should he so want.

The underlying philosophy of yoga is best introduced little by little. It becomes absorbed almost indirectly, unconsciously — until the teacher starts to hear it 'coming back' from members of the class as if the ideas were their own! At that point it can be taught more directly. The higher the intelligence rating of those in the class, the more they will take to it — then yoga becomes the whole way of life, and is not just practised for its more obvious practical, physical values.

Mental Handicap

The difficulties that require special consideration when dealing with mentally handicapped people are excess energy, difficulty in following the spoken word, and difficulty in concentrating for any length of time. These are the normal teaching problems for any teacher of mentally handicapped people. The excess energy can be dealt with by allowing a certain amount of rampaging about, 'blowing off steam', before the class starts. This should be followed by the usual period of 'collecting into oneself', then concentration on breathing—first the relaxed breathing, then the breathing of action. In the latter, full use of all possible arm and leg movements should be made. A really vigorous warming up session should follow, with plenty of movements that involve all four limbs: such as drumming with the hands on the thighs, and the heels on the floor at the same time, if sitting down; a good deal of rolling if lying; or plenty of running on the spot with arm circling at the same time if standing. See Chapter Three.

If all this has been vigorous enough there should be no problem over the main body of the lesson. But it is as well not to try to hold any posture for long—variety retains interest. Consequently use more than the usual number of postures in a session for mentally handicapped pupils.

It will be found that members of this class react better to a demonstrated posture than to a wordy description of it. The posture should be demonstrated in stages if necessary, and each step checked on before moving on to the next, but without long delays. Consequently it is a good idea for the teacher to have one or two helpers.

Mentally handicapped people are often stiff and are likely to be uncoordinated. Initially they may require a good deal of physical help, and concentration on very simple postures. But there is no reason why they should not ultimately reach a high standard. As they improve it is as well to progress to the more complicated postures, because they can quickly get bored with what appears to them to be easy, and a waste of time! Lavish encouragement and praise is part of any teacher's routine in dealing with such a class—that, and brightness and fun, are essential. Any yoga class should have laughter in it, even more so when the pupils are mentally handicapped.

At the end of the class, the relaxation should not be too long — but if the session has been well organised, there should be no trouble over five minutes or so. The time without any accompanying speech needs to be kept short — 'recognition of sounds' is a useful starter, see series two, number 3) in Chapter Ten, particularly if there are plenty of sounds to be heard in the building. The post-relaxation 'wake up' needs more than one good stretch, and perhaps another roll or two.

This is also a good time to try to draw out some feed back — which helps the teacher to keep well in touch with the class and their likes and dislikes. All comments should be welcomed, and perhaps developed somewhat by the teacher — this satisfies the pupil, makes the others more prepared to be articulate in their turn, and enables the teacher to deal with such irrelevancies as may be produced.

All that has been said in this chapter is meant to allow for a great deal of variation: according to the individual's age, what he is like as a person, the type of handicap (physical, mental or emotional), the degree of the handicap, and his general circumstances, as well as the personality of the teacher and the kind of help available. Yoga is a tailor-made activity, tailored to fit the individual, and herein lies its great potential for handicapped people. It can be carried out at their pace, suited to their own angle, in line with their particular disability, and the mode of approach can be adapted for each and every individual.

3: General Principles and Preliminaries

Yoga postures have evolved over centuries to exercise all the muscles, to 'work on' the viscera, and to stimulate the endocrine glands, the brain and the voluntary and involuntary nervous systems. They also work at a mental level, conquering tension, producing tranquillity and serenity, calming and disciplining the mind. Practice, if persevering, results in a high level of health, a body maintained free of disease, and a mind that is clear and controlled.

General Principles for Working on Postures
The best time for practising is in the morning, after washing and teeth cleaning and before breaking one's fast. (This would also be a good—but unlikely—time for a class!) Even before this, the day can have been greeted with some breathing exercises and general stretching of arms and legs in bed (see spine stretching exercises on page 36).

Otherwise, a good time is during the evening. Postures are often found to be easier during the evening, as the body stiffens up overnight, through lying still.

The first important thing is to find a quiet spot where one is unlikely to be disturbed. To practise out of doors is ideal but usually impracticable, particularly if a physical handicap is involved. The clothing worn for practising should be scant and light, leaving all movements free, yet warm enough. Cold inhibits movement, so there is no point in trying to be hardy! It is good to have a yoga mat to practise on, but any rug or folded blanket will serve. Whatever is used it should be kept for one's personal use and for yoga alone.

A Few Physical Reminders
It is impossible to do yoga on a full stomach. There should be a gap of three hours at the very least after a heavy meal, two hours after a light meal and getting on for an hour—at the

very least half an hour—after a drink. Anybody disbelieving this is soon convinced if he tries to practise after a shorter interval!

Again it is not possible to practise yoga with a full bladder—it should be emptied just before starting, and during a class or practice session if necessary. People with stomas and bags—e.g. people with spina bifida having ileal loop bladders—should be advised that their urine flow will greatly increase during the class or practice, so they should empty their appliances just before they start.

A full rectum too makes for very uncomfortable yoga practice. A bowel action before a period of work at a class or practice should be encouraged. A really distended gut makes yoga impossible.

Some people find yoga work difficult on the first day of a period, even for two or three days if the normal flow is heavy. The more strenuous postures may stimulate the flow to an uncomfortable degree, and this seems more noticeable when tampons are worn. People do not need to miss out on their yoga work, but to take it at a leisurely pace, to do each posture fewer times, to hold for a shorter time, and to avoid inverted postures. Relaxation is markedly beneficial in spasmodic dysmenorrhoea: all the postures that increase abdominal circulation can help to relieve dysmenorrhoea of the congestive type.

Pre-warming up

On first contact with the class it is a good idea to tell everybody to 'draw back' into himself, 'collect' himself as a whole person, and then just 'watch the breath'. For this the eyes should be closed. This may or may not induce relaxation, but it certainly helps towards concentration. The pupil should 'watch', 'observe' his own breath coming in and going out, and watch the process get slower and gentler, expiration always being longer than inspiration. Breathing should quieten down until the only movement is a gentle rise of the abdomen, if lying down, or forward movement if in a chair, on breathing in; and the reverse on breathing out. It helps a great deal if the teacher stresses that breathing out is the important movement, and that breathing in is unimportant. It will happen anyway if the pupil pauses after breathing out—sooner or later air just starts to be drawn back into the lungs, without any definite effort, when the body needs it. In the early stages of yoga with handicapped people, the acquisition of this relaxed and effortless breathing may take literally hours of work — in short stints, needless to say.

The next task is to learn to relax, to let go, and to combine complete bodily relaxation with the breathing of relaxation. The teacher instructs as follows:

> Lie in the floor posture, spine straight, head in a straight line with the body, shoulders turned slightly outwards, arms a little away from the body, and legs turned out at hips, knees and ankles relaxed so that the feet fall slightly outwards.
>
> Let all tension drain out of the body.
>
> Tense the muscles of the face, screwing up eyes and mouth — then let them all go loose.
>
> Tighten the muscles of the neck, lifting the head off the floor — let it relax back on to the floor.
>
> Tighten the muscles round the shoulder girdle, lifting the shoulders off the floor — let them go loose and settle back again.
>
> Extend the arms, lift them stiffly off the floor — drop them and let them go loose.
>
> Ball the fists up tight — loosen them.
>
> Contract the muscles of the abdomen hard, drawing them in against the spine — then let them relax.
>
> Contract the muscles of the buttocks hard — relax them.
>
> Tighten the thighs, pulling the kneecaps up as far as possible — relax them.
>
> Extend the lower legs, lifting them off the ground — let them relax and sink back.
>
> Push the toes as far away from the trunk as possible — let them relax.
>
> Try to maintain the body in this totally relaxed position while working on the relaxed breath.
>
> Check various areas at intervals!

Next, before proceeding to any postures, there must be some 'action breaths'. It may help to let the pupil start by breathing in through the mouth for this, until the practical difference between the relaxed breath and an action breath is established in his mind. For the 'action' breath the abdomen is held firm, not rigid, the shoulders are kept down, but not with any strain, and there is a larger intake of air — consequently the ribs move upwards and outwards, as is usually said, like the top of a bucket. It is easy enough to 'feel' with the hands what the ribs do, placing them on the lower ribs.

The next step is for the arms to be brought into play, extending the action breath still further (see Chapter Four). Then there should be a return to the relaxed breath for a moment or two, before starting on the warming up routine.

Warming up
This is a very important part of any yoga class — it gets the circulation going and the muscles warmed and prepared for action. It is a vital necessity therefore for the physically handicapped. The value lies in movement — no matter how ragged, how uncoordinated. For the young, the emotionally taut, the mentally handicapped, it can be a means of letting off steam, after which the pupil is more prepared to concentrate, to attempt to control the action of his limbs, to work with slow dignity, thinking of every action as he performs it. Three different routines are listed below, with details following.

Standing Routine
   Finger movement
   Wrist movement
   Forearm flick
   Whole arm movements
   Ankle and leg rotation
   Leg swinging
   Spine flexion
   Lateral flexion
   Trunk rotation
   Hip movement
   Walking and running on the spot
   'Ha' Breaths, three or four times

Chair routine, or sitting on the floor
   Finger movement
   Wrist movement
   Forearm flick

Whole arm movement
Toe pull
Leg extension
Walking upstairs
Rag doll breath

Floor routine — lying down
Finger movement
Wrist movement
Forearm flick
Whole arm movement
Toe Pull
Leg separation
Drumming
Rolling

A *Standing routine*

1   Screw the fists up, then loosen — extending the fingers widely. Repeat 3 or 4 times.
2   Flick hands from the wrist, as if shaking drops of water off for a duration of 20 seconds.
3   Flick the arms from the elbow downwards, including the wrist flick. Tuck elbows well into the sides.
4   Raise the arms from the shoulder up over the head, then drop loosely, allowing to swing freely.
5   Extend the arms horizontally and rotate in one piece, first forwards and then backwards, making the rotatory movement into wider and wider circles.
6   Stand on one leg and lift the other, rotating the foot at the ankle, first clockwise and then anticlockwise. Repeat with the other leg.
7   Stand on one leg, lift the other and rotate the leg at the knee, first clockwise then anticlockwise. Repeat with the other leg.
8   Stand on one leg and swing the other diagonally across the body, making as wide a movement as possible. Repeat this with the other leg.
9   Stand with the feet 500 mm (18″) apart, fold the arms loosely behind the back and bend partly backwards, breathing in. Return to the upright position then bend forward, breathing out, and extend the arms forward at

shoulder level, pulling the head back. Hollow the back and breathe normally for 30–60 seconds. Then drop hands, arms and trunk forward towards the floor on another exhalation, bending the knees slightly. Return to starting position on an inhalation.

10   Stand with the feet 500 mm (18″) apart, toes pointing straight forward. Raise the arms to shoulder level sideways. Then bend sideways on an exhalation, to the right, bringing the left arm up to point directly toward the ceiling. Hold the position, breathing normally, for 50–60 seconds. Return to the standing position on an inhalation and perform the posture on the other side.

11   Stand with the feet 500 mm (18″) apart and, moving from the waist, rotate the arms and trunk, first round one way, then round the other, breathing normally. Do not hurry.

12   a) Standing with feet 500 mm (18″) apart, roll or jerk the right hip outwards, then the left hip, then reverse (a fairly rapid movement from side to side). Repeat 4 times.
b) Circular movement first with right hip, then with left.
c) Rotate both hips together, as if using a hula-hoop.

13   Walk, then run on the spot — start with just coming on to the toe, i.e. with neither foot leaving the ground, proceed to walk, one foot off the ground, and then to run, both feet off the ground together. Either get faster and faster, with the feet only just leaving the floor, or gradually raise the knees higher and higher.

14   Perform several 'Ha' breaths (see Chapter Four).

B *Sitting routine* — in chair, wheelchair, or on the floor.
1, 2, 3, 4, and 5 above are possible, though for those sitting on the floor the hands will just come down on to the floor in 4 and not swing freely.

6   Instead of 6 above, pull toes up towards knee, then push down and away. Repeat 3 or 4 times.

7   Part the legs as widely as possible, then bring them sharply together again. Repeat 3 or 4 times.

8   'Walk upstairs', one step at a time, as rapidly as possible, i.e. raise first one leg, then the other, either bending at the knees or raising from the buttocks. Knees may be flexed or straight.

9   Drum with the heels on the floor or footrest, then add drumming with the hands on the thighs at the same time — reach as much speed as possible even if the limbs are very uncoordinated.

10 Perform several 'Ha' breaths, collapsing forward at the waist on expiration like a rag doll (see Chapter Four).

C *Lying Routine*

1, 2, 3, 4, 5, as in A. In 4, the arms can be taken right over the head to the floor behind.

6, 7, 8, 9, as in B.

10 Hold hands together, and roll, using the lower part of the body as a weight to push the whole body over once or twice in one direction off the yoga mat, and then back on to it. This last is of particular value for a physically handicapped person who rarely uses every part of the body at the same time.

Mentally handicapped people can all do these simple exercises, by imitation. Rolling is particularly popular.

Physically handicapped pupils may require help, according to the degree of handicap: a paralysed limb may be worked by somebody else, fingers can be spread out, arm lifted, toes lifted, legs separated etc. Much help may be necessary with rolling, particularly to start with, before pupils learn the secret of using the weight of the bottom half of the body to topple them over, by sheer mechanics.

The warming up is of value even if *most* of the movements have been carried out by somebody else: indeed sometimes it pays to have a helper to help even with movements that the pupil can achieve alone, in order that he may do them faster, and so stimulate the circulation. On the other hand, with elderly people, warming up must not be so strenuous that they become exhausted before the yoga exercises proper begin (see Elderly People, Chapter Eight).

Post Warming Up

After the warming up process, and before proceeding to the regular postures, there are some preliminary exercises to do, some of which stretch the spine and some of which further release tension, allowing a free flow of energy through the body. Each involves the breath of action. It is a good idea to perform one or two of them: this, coupled with the breathing work, ensures that there is ample energy present for the work that is to follow. More are not necessary, unless a very long yoga session is planned. This is rare with handicapped classes.

Some preliminaries to postures
Except for number one, these are not possible in wheelchairs or chairs.

1 SPINE STRETCHING
   a Lie on the floor, inhale, stretch the right arm over the head and the right leg out straight as far as possible, on the outbreath. Then relax. Repeat with the left arm and left leg. Then repeat both three times.
   b Inhale, stretch the right arm over the head and the left leg out straight as far as possible, on the outbreath. Then relax. Repeat with the left arm and right leg. Then repeat both three times.
2 In a sitting position, with legs stretched out in front, lift the leg—if possible—and walk on buttocks some ten 'paces' forward and return. Repeat this once. This can be done as a shuffle without lifting the leg first.
3 Lying on the back, inhale and draw the right knee on to the chest, while extending the left leg as far as possible on an outbreath: return right leg to starting position and relax left leg. Change legs. Repeat cycle 3 times.
4 *Of particular value for the physically handicapped.* (An exercise which may prove extremely difficult). Lying on the back, sit up by means of rolling on to the right shoulder and right elbow, and pushing off; when sitting fully erect, lie down by rolling on to the left elbow and then the left shoulder and finally on to the back. Repeat in the other direction—i.e. on to the left shoulder and elbow to get up, and the right elbow and shoulder to go down. Repeat the whole cycle the other way round.
5 Sit with the legs outstretched, then bend the knees, bringing the feet in towards the buttocks. Pass the arms under the thighs and clasp the elbows on the outbreath, then slide the feet forward, keeping the chest close to the knees. Return to starting position on an inhalation.

2 These can be performed by people sitting on chairs or in wheelchairs, as well as seated on the floor, provided the chair does not have high arms (some wheelchair arms come out), and the pupil can sit fairly far forward.

   a Sit with legs outstretched, clench fists and lean as far forward as possible, breathing out; then breathe in and lean as far back as possible, bringing the fists to the chest as in rowing. The pull should be felt on the abdominal muscles. Repeat 10 times.

   b Clench fists in front of chest, elbows bent, make circling movements with the arms, first leaning forwards, then backwards, then turning to the right and to the left in both the backward and the forward position.

   c With arms at full stretch, move them alternately up and down as if pulling a rope. Breathe evenly throughout.

Posture Work

A full yoga posture sequence should not be attempted until these preliminaries have taken place — that is, recollection, breathing of relaxation, action breaths, warming up exercises, and, if desired, one or two post-warming up exercises. This is particularly important for physically handicapped people who start with such poor circulations, and are almost always 'out of condition'.

There are certain principles that the pupil should then try to keep in mind throughout, because if mental preparation is correct, the value of each posture is enhanced. These are:

1 First relax and visualise the pose as it should be — complete and perfect. Think of the type of pose it is, and what it is meant to achieve for the body.

2 'Think down into' the muscles what it is they are about to do: visualise the limbs as being capable of free-flowing movements (this is particularly important for handicapped people, who should not think of their own inadequacies).

3 Coordinate the breath with bodily movements: that is, begin the movement just *after* inspiration, or expiration starts, according to the type of movement (most movements are on the outbreath), and finish the movement just before the breath ends.

4   The general breathing rule to follow is: exhale for folding up or closing movements; inhale for opening out or extension movements.

5   Also coordinate the brain with the body, thinking through each part of any movement as it is undertaken, still keeping the complete, perfect picture in the mind.

6   Observe yourself throughout, that is before starting, then during the movements, while going into and on coming out of the pose, *and* also after finishing.

7   Stop both the movement and the hold before there is any strain, but work at the posture all the time it is being held. Beginners will rarely exceed a minute. Whilst the posture is being held, breathing should be deep, balanced and through the nose, (Listening to the breathing that is going on quickly tells the teacher that the pose has been held for long enough!)

8   Move slowly both into *and* out of the posture, remembering that the intermediate stages are as important as the final ones. Indeed it may be only the half-way stages that physically handicapped people can reach.

9   Constantly check for relaxation — muscles shorten in tension, whereas they lengthen in relaxation, and it is then often possible to move a little further into the posture. Face, neck, eye muscles, which are little involved in most postures, can be relaxed throughout.

10 Do not indulge in any competition — not even with yourself. Make no comparisons with how you did the same pose yesterday.

Every posture in a sequence will promote the circulation in one or several areas, and will stimulate the viscera, the glands and both nervous systems, No violence or speed should be used — postures work of themselves, and a slow pace is essential it they are to be effective. Slowness in action coupled with the right mental attitudes and proper use of the breath make for rapid progress. In every pose the pupil must let his body give in to gravity. Every posture should be followed by a counter-pose — that is, if the spine or trunk has been bent one way, then in the next posture the bend should be the other way. This is very important in order to ensure fully balanced development.

The gradual acquisition of power to achieve a movement,

and of control over such power so that the movement is both slow and smooth, is of incalculable value for a handicapped person. Simple postures are the most necessary ones, and even in these the intermediate stages are just as important as the end results.

Combinations of Movement (These may have to be varied to take account of physical handicap).

Most postures are combinations of two or more of the four basic movements which are: backward bend, forward bend, sideways bend, and lastly, twisting. In a normal session, postures are usually worked into a sequence as follows:

1 Standing, with forward and sideways bending;
2 Lying, a recuperation from standing — bending both forwards and backwards;
3 Inverted, coming when both 1, and 2, have prepared for this, and when all the muscles are warm and stretched;
4 Backwards bending — to offset the forward bend;
5 Twisting;
6 Forward bending again, concluding with this, it being the range of movements with which the body is most familiar.

The whole sequence in any class or practice is orientated towards stretching, twisting or balancing (using the power of the retained breath with more experienced pupils, see Chapter Four), finishing with a stretch. For each of the four basic movements there are some postures that are very simple, and that can be tackled with almost any degree of disability, and others that are progressively more difficult. Standing positions are deceptive, and even simple ones are 'strong', that is they require a good physique. They should be used sparingly with elderly people, will be out of the question for many handicapped people and must be kept of short duration for children (see Chapter Two).

Modification of postures
This is essential with disability. Quite often, apart from the specific disability and any non-functioning arm or arms and/or leg or legs, the body is generally unfit. It has probably been consistently under-exercised: a physically handicapped

person may never have had any exertion to exercise the heart muscle, has never moved or run fast to stimulate deep breathing. Such people are also particularly prone to stress and tension, because of their general physical problems, and their difficulties in coping mentally, emotionally and financially.

Unfitness, as well as many disabilities, causes poor co-ordination and induces restricted breathing — resulting in still more tension; frequently too, handicapped people are over-weight, due to bad feeding and lack of exercise; or conversely, because of fatigue, poor muscle or other feeding difficulties, they are undernourished — which can be combined with being overweight. In either case they lack strength. Many areas of the body are stiff, notably the spine, or flabby and weak — even paralysed. There may be grossly impaired control due to athetoid movements, tremor, etc.

As a consequence of one, more, or all of these factors, the full posture is very often not possible and must be modified, and minimal movement accepted. For example many spastics cannot sit up straight on the floor with the legs stretched out flat on the floor in front: as soon as the spine is straightened and the head lifted up, they fall over backwards. Consequently, the starting point for the back stretch is quite different from that for someone without a handicap.

To give another example, people with spina bifida have no 'weight' in the bottom part of the body, and so cannot make use of the force of gravity, nor use their legs as an anchor on which to pivot.

A spastic youngster with ceaseless athetoid movements may have a resting respiratory rate in the thirties, so it may take him a complete session to relax in any way.

Modifications are fully treated in the posture Chapters, Five, Six and Seven. Sequence variations are to be found in Chapter Eight.

4: Pranayama, Breath Control

Pranayama is the science of breath control. The word 'ayama' means 'to control'. But 'prana' is far more than the breath. Prana is the sum total of cosmic energy. It is present in air — yet not one of its constituent gases; present in food and water — yet not one of these substances; present in sunlight — yet neither warmth nor ultraviolet light. Prana is taken in to the body in all of these — but chiefly in air.

In yoga we believe that this prana, this energy, can be stored in the nervous system, for example in the solar plexus, and can then be directed through the body at will. These concepts seem remote from the simple breathing exercises, the basic and elementary breath control contained in this chapter, but the goal of yoga may be defined as twofold: combining control of the mind with control of this vital energy, which has been collected and stored within the body. Consequently the postures detailed in the next three chapters, and the simple breathing procedures in this, are working together in their different ways towards the same aim.

Therefore prana, the life breath, is considerably more than the taking in of necessary oxygen from inspired air. It is the vital force in every being, pervading everything. Air is the most essential of all 'foods'. Better breathing means a better supply of prana, that is a better supply of energy.

Breathing deeply and well has to be relearned, for this innate skill is quickly lost in childhood. There is a world of difference between breathing shallowly and incorrectly, and breathing for health and vitality, tapping a store of infinite energy. Prana is also the healer: diseases do not gain a hold on a body that is totally permeated with pranic energy. Slow deep rhythmic breathing denotes a mind calm, contented, relaxed — and not only does it denote it, it also *produces* it. A breathing pattern made up of short shallow jerks shows a mind full of fear, tension, anxiety. Moreover it can augment these stresses in the mind.

Excitement or emotional stress in the mind affects the breathing *rate*, while tension affects the *depth* of breathing. With emotion the rate is quicker, with tension the breathing is shallower. Deliberate regulation of the breathing, that is slowing and deepening it, calms the emotions and relieves tension — consequently the first task in yoga is that of regulating the breathing. Relaxation stems from this. But there is much more to it than that — breathing therapy marks the beginning of mind control. Focussing the attention on the breath is one means of securing 'one-pointedness' of mind. Moreover a rhythmic pattern of breathing, slow, deep and steady, strengthens the respiratory system itself.

With anyone who is emotionally unbalanced and in a state of inner conflict, the physiological approach to these problems by means of breath control is a great help. It strongly reinforces the psychological approach. In fatigue situations, respiration can be increased in depth, and the energy of the breath directed into any 'sleepy' areas, to invigorate them.

Anatomically speaking there are two kinds of breathing: external and internal.

1 *External* breathing takes place in the lungs. The organs concerned include the nostrils, nasal passages, respiratory muscles, bronchi and bronchioles and the diaphragm, as well as the nervous and chemical mechanisms necessary to enable air to reach the lungs in the first place. Their action, drawing in air rich in oxygen, and expelling air filled with carbon dioxide, depends upon an efficiently working diaphragm. The diaphragm is pulled down on inspiration, and so the lungs *expand*. Most breathing is automatic — controlled by the carbon dioxide level in the blood. But it can also, to a certain extent, be consciously controlled.

2 *Internal*, or cellular, breathing takes place across cell membranes throughout the entire body. Red blood corpuscles, carrying oxygen they have taken up in the lungs, release this, taking up carbon dioxide in return. Breath control aims particularly at stimulating this second kind of breathing, assisted by the stimulation of the circulation effected by the postures.

It follows then that yogic breath control operates at several levels. It raises the level of general health, by providing a supply of richly oxygenated blood; provides a strong reserve of energy, that can be called upon at will; calms the mind; tones the nervous system; and clarifies awareness, thus preparing the way for meditation. Consequently it may be termed a physical means towards a mental, emotional and spiritual end.

Breathing exercises must be practised regularly, with as much seriousness of purpose as the postures. They need never become dull and boring, because they can be so widely varied. The teacher should aim for some degree of relaxation in her pupils before starting work on breathing. Beginners always have a tendency to tense up before starting a breathing programme. 'Awareness' of the breath should be cultivated—it is a concept of value in meditation (see Chapter Ten).

Postures in yoga can be of little use until the proper working of the diaphragm is to some extent restored. When the diaphragm is functioning to capacity, the resultant correct oxygenation of the blood allows the functioning of the whole body to be regulated. Severe handicap is greatly helped by improved natural breathing, for poor oxygenation and poor circulation are a frequent concomitant of severe handicap.

The aim of controlled breathing in yogic postures is to maintain a harmony between the movement of the body and the movement of the breath. Expanding movements are made on inhalation, that is the chest and abdomen expand when the body as a whole is opening out. By the same principle contracting movements are made on inhalation. Twisting movements are usually made on exhalation, for in them the body exerts a restricting pressure, which helps to empty the lungs. Some other movements—for example leg raising—also take place during exhalation because the movement of the legs has a contracting effect upon the abdomen. (if this movement were done during inhalation there would be conflict between the downward pressure on the diaphragm and the contraction of the abdomen.)

Not only rate and depth, but also the quality of the breathing has an effect upon movement and posture—it should be even and refined. The synchronisation of breathing and movement encourages concentration.

As we said in the previous chapter, the breath starts just

before the movement, and finishes just after it. Consequently the duration of the breath ultimately decides the speed of the movement.

Retention of breath stimulates cellular breathing—the second type. The ability to retain depends not upon taking a deep breath, as might be imagined, but upon the previous two or three deep complete breaths—for these will have increased the volume of oxygen held in the blood. If retention takes place after about five deep breaths, the last one having been the slower one which passed into retention, and if, while these breaths are taking place the mind focusses on bodily functions, then the heartbeat will be found to be slowed. Retention should always be followed by a slow exhalation with a forced end, i.e. pulling in of the rib cage and then a smooth transition to ordinary breathing.

Remember that 'The wise man breathes with his head', that is, breathing requires concentration and thought.

When the breath is held, the system stores energy, and more waste matters are lost from the cells, because cellular respiration is still going on. If the expulsion following retention is quick, then the stored energy is released, but if it is slow, then energy is retained (in the solar plexus) and only the waste products are lost.

The student should remember that bending forward on expiration makes use of the force of gravity to help the expiration, as in 'ha' breath, or on going into the Dog pose from lying flat.

When sitting for these exercises, the pupil can drop his chin into the sternal notch and close his eyes. The arms should be relaxed, hands on knees, and the thumb and little finger approximated.

The pupil must not exceed his own capacity/cycle; there must be no force, no strain. Even breathing means even temper. Space of time should be allowed between breathing and the carrying out of postures, longer if the breathing comes before the postures, ten minutes if the postures precede the breathing. These are counsels for later on, and more advanced work, and are not so necessary to be observed in the early days of short lessons. Ideally the student should relax into the floor pose, and should always 'switch off' after breath control exercises for five to ten minutes.

The average respiratory rate (of the ordinary person) at rest is 15 per minute. It increases with indigestion, pain, fever, cold, cough, emotion; and it is also frequently much higher in people with a physical handicap.

Breathing exercises sometimes demand a specific number of counts for inhalation, retention, exhalation and pausing. But concentrating on this may produce tension; and any over-effort at retention is harmful, and must be avoided. Retention varies with the postures — retained breath gives the surge of energy which needs to be employed for extra effort, but it must not be practised until the pupil is proficient in rhythmic inhalation and exhalation.

Exhalation can be a) slow, deliberate and long drawn out, or b) rapid and abrupt. The first is the type used in relaxation, where it must always be longer than inhalation. This type of exhalation can be carried out with wide open mouth and dropped shoulders. It is a real safety valve: slow well-controlled exhalations are very useful in labour, or preceding times of stress such as competitions, interviews or exams, or just before making a stage entrance; b) is self-explanatory.

The *pause* following exhalation can vary from a couple of seconds to 20 or 30 seconds. It slows breathing overall, and also slows the heart rate. It calms in over-excitement.

Some General Rules for Breathing Practice
This should not be carried out too close to a meal.

The first essential is an easy position, freeing the thorax. The student must be relaxed before starting breathing practice, and must remain relaxed throughout. (This will need checking on at intervals. Students are always prone to tense their legs and arms as they try to concentrate.)

The length of inhalation or exhalation must never be forced — there should be no great *effort* towards breathing more slowly. The breath must be relaxed and comfortable, then it will lengthen naturally.

The breath must also never be held for long periods.

Loose clothing is a must for breathing practice, as is good ventilation. Where possible it is a good idea to carry out breathing practice outdoors. Washing the face and hands, and gargling, makes a good start. The nostrils should be cleared by preliminary blowing. Breathing exercises must be pleasant—the pupil should be told to stop as soon as discomfort or strain arises.

Sequences of exercises

Four different sequences of breathing exercises follow. (The same exercise will be found more than once.)
They are:

A Sequence of breathing exercises when lying down
B Sequence of exercises when confined to a chair
C Sequence of exercises making use of a standing position
D Traditional pranayama

As a rough guide, the exercises in A, B and C serve when breathing exercises form part of a normal yoga session. (Indeed all sessions should start with the relaxed breath and action breath of A and C.) The exercises of D are useful when a whole session is given over to breathing work.

A   *Simple Sequence of breathing exercises, lying on the floor*

a)   RELAXED BREATH

The student lies in the Floor pose (for details of pose see Chapter Five). Attention should be focussed on the breath; as the pupil breathes in the abdomen rises, as he breathes out the abdomen falls. The breathing has to be quite unforced, both effortless and soundless. Breathing out is the more positive movement and is longer, breathing in is 'unimportant'. The pupil can be told that if he pauses after breathing out, at a given point, when the body needs it, air will 'sneak' or 'float' in.

The face is smooth and relaxed, shoulders loose, chest quite 'floppy'. The only thing moving is the abdomen, and that is not a deliberate pushing out or pulling in, but the result of the air inside coming and going.

b)   THE BREATH OF ACTION—REVITALISING BREATH

Still in the Floor pose, the pupil changes his manner of breathing in. On breathing in, the ribs move outwards and upwards with as wide a movement as possible. This action breath involves a very positive intake of air. The abdomen is held firmly, but not rigidly, until most of the air is out, when it is drawn in and backwards towards the spine. Beginners

may be helped to master this type of breathing by taking one
or two breaths through the mouth at first, but once the rib
movement and abdominal position have been grasped the
mouth should be kept closed throughout — both inhalation
and exhalation taking place through the nose. There may be
a sound in the throat, on both inhalation and exhalation: 'Sa'
on inspiration, 'Ha' on expiration.

These two types of breathing must be practised until the
student can go from one to the other and back again without
effort, and with full confidence. Once this is the case, a whole
series of arm movements can be married in with b):

1 The arms move in time with the breath, being raised up
over the front of the body to touch the floor beyond the
head on inspiration, and placed back down at the sides
on expiration. Helpers move the arms if need be.

Where breathing is rapid — as in most spastic
people — the arms can move up a little way on inspiration, stay stationary for the expiration, move again on
the next inhalation, stay stationary on expiration
again — and so on, perhaps taking four or five breath
cycles to reach the floor behind the head. Then the
reverse takes place coming back — the arms move on
expiration and stay stationary on inhalation. After a
spell of this the pupil should revert to the relaxed
breathing again.

2 Next, the student can combine the breath of action with
head turning; that is, he turns the head to the left on
inhalation, and then lets it drift back to the centre on
exhalation; then he repeats this to the right. He should
revert to the breathing of relaxation again after five or
six breaths of this type.

3 Then the student can lift the head to look at the feet on
the in breath, and let it drop back on the out breath.
Again he should revert to a) after five or six breaths.

4 Next, as well as turning the head as in 2, he should
gently roll the whole arm outwards at the shoulder,
down to the fingers, and roll the leg out from the hip in
the same way, on inspiration, then let them both move
slowly back on exhalation. The head should move to the
right and the arm and leg to the left, and then vice

versa — in short, a mini-stretch. He reverts to a) again after some five or six breaths of this type.

5   On the in breath, the student slides on to the top of the head by contracting the neck muscles and raising the chin, then he slips back into a normal position on expiration. He reverts to a) again after five or six breaths.

6   The student lies with the feet placed comfortably flat on the floor, fairly near the buttocks, then tenses thighs and buttocks on the in breath, and relaxes on the out breath, reverting to a) as before. 5 and 6 can be combined.

7   The next step is as in 6, except that the buttocks as well as being tensed are lifted off the ground on inspiration, and lowered again on expiration. As usual, the student reverts to a) after five or six breaths of this type.

8   Finally the student performs 7, but he extends the 'lift-off' to include the trunk, so that the body is now balanced on the feet and shoulders. The buttocks and thighs must be completely relaxed on expiration in all these exercises, that is 6, 7 and 8. After five or six breaths he reverts to a).

9   In this variation the student lies with the legs out-stretched and the heels pushed well down away from the trunk, on inspiration. On expiration he draws one flexed knee up on to his chest, and on inspiration puts it back down, repeating with the other leg. Finally he draws both flexed knees up together — expiration accompanies the legs moving up on to the abdomen, and inspiration the downwards straightening. The chin is brought over to meet the knees too. The student reverts to a) as usual, after completing three rounds of this. The arms can be clasped round the knee or knees if desired.

10 Action breath in a 'towards the plough' position:
    a) Lie with the legs outstretched, then on expiration draw the feet up and place near the buttocks;
    b) Breathe in, then on expiration draw the knees up on to the chest, thighs close to abdomen;
    c) Breathe in, then on expiration extend the legs at the knee, and lift the bottom off the floor, using the

hands to help if necessary—until the feet are above the head;

d) Breathe evenly in this position for five or six breaths;

e) Revert to the starting position, moving on inhalation and pausing on exhalation.

Apart from their use at the beginning of a yoga session—where it is envisaged that a few out of the ten would be practised—ten to fifteen minutes spent practising these exercises on their own is an excellent therapy, particularly for people with little muscle left. Just two or three combined with simple stretches, as found in Chapter Five, also form an excellent 'yogic start' to the day, loosening and providing energy. If need be a helper can help with the limb movements. All of them can be performed in bed and could provide material for a pre-yoga course for a week or so.

It should be noted that the in breath is fairly swift once the impulse comes, in action breathing, whereas the out breath is slow and controlled. There must be no painful effort in either direction.

B *Sequence in a seated position* (chair, backless stool or wheelchair)

Both the relaxed breath a) and the breath of action b) can be carried out perfectly well when seated, even in a wheelchair. It is very important to have the spine as straight as possible, and the head straight with the spine. For relaxed breathing the abdomen moves gently outwards on inspiration. The raising of the arms can be introduced in just the same way as when lying down, as can the tightening of the muscles of thighs and buttocks.

Turning of the head to one side with an eversion of one arm from the shoulders downwards on the other side on inspiration is another modification.

An exercise of particular value for people confined to wheelchairs is to lean well forward on expiration, thus putting pressure on the gut. This movement should take place while breathing out with the mouth open. If it is 'assisted' by a compression of the abdomen, as in forced expiration, the whole procedure is particularly useful against constipation as it raises the intra-abdominal pressure. It also helps to change the unchanging air usually static in the lung bases.

Following a) and b) there are a considerable number of breathing exercises that can be carried out while seated:

1   Breathing in time with a particular sound—such as following the heart beat for in and out. (This should not be carried out for long as it is too rapid; a clock tick may serve better.)

2   Breathing in naturally, but out each time to a count of one, then out each time to a count of two, of three, etc., rising to as many as possible—even ten!

3   Taking a full breath while raising the shoulder towards the ears on inspiration, with the glottis half closed, —the resultant sound in the throat shows the smoothness or otherwise of the intake. This is a means of acquiring instant vitality and may also help to clear a mood of depression or irritation.

4   The Bellows breath. Rapid breathing, equal in *and* out, with a duration of one second each, perhaps *slightly* longer on the in breath. The abdomen should be smartly pulled in on expiration. With this type of breathing there may possibly be slight giddiness at first. This breath must never be forced and speed should not be aimed at. A cycle of between five and ten rounds is sufficient, one round being both 'in' and 'out'.

5   a) *One-nostril breathing*
     In this, inhalation and exhalation should be of the same length. The pupil inhales on the right side and exhales on the left side for about ten cycles, and then reverses, closing the other nostril with two fingers.

     b) *Alternate nostril breathing*
     This balances the right and left sides of the body, and induces tranquillity. It can be performed for eight to ten cycles, one cycle being:
     i) in through the right nostril with the left closed;
     ii) out through the left nostril with the right closed;
     iii)in again through the left nostril with the right still closed;
     iv) finally exhale through the right nostril with the left nostril closed.
     The position should be held by means of the right thumb closing the right nostril, the first and second

fingers on the forehead, and the third and fourth fingers closing the left nostril.

Inhalation and exhalation on each side should be of the same length. There must be no pause made after exhalation, until the pupil can manage to pause after inhalation. The adjustment of the pressure exercised on the nostrils governs the rate of inhalation and exhalation. Tension must be avoided — it can occur very easily in this exercise.

c) The Bellows breath can be repeated using only one nostril, first the right with the left closed, then the left with the right closed, for ten cycles, then take a slow deep breath.

As a general rule, people who have to remain seated can achieve fewer active postures than those who lie, consequently in their sessions rather more time can be given over to breathing exercises.

C *Exercise sequence, standing, involving the use of active postures*

The student stands in the Erect posture (for posture description see Chapter Five), performs a) and b) as in A on page 46, then proceeds to the use of the arms, as follows:

1 *The Simple 'Ha' breath*
   The student stands with the feet 400–500mm (15″–18″) apart. On breathing in he raises the arms above the head, and leans slightly backwards from the hips, then, on breathing out collapses forward, loose at hips and waist, exhaling an audible 'Ha', with head dropped, arms loose and swinging freely from the shoulders, hands at floor level, mouth open. The knees can bend. The student repeats this whole breath three times. He then reverts to a) for several breaths — that is the breathing of relaxation, in this instance carried out standing erect, unless he intends to proceed to exercise 2 below.

2 The 'Ha' breath is repeated as above, but when at floor level, the student places his right hand in the centre of the back at hip level, with the palm uppermost; then the

left hand ditto. He then pulls the shoulder blades together. He lifts the chin and comes up on a further inspiration, relaxing into the Erect posture on expiration.

Both 1 and 2 are repeated in this way, three times, then the student reverts to a), that is relaxed breathing for several breaths.

3 Next he interlocks his hands behind the back and leans back on an inspiration, pulling the shoulders well together and raising the arms behind him. Hands, shoulders and arms all return to their normal position on expiration. After doing this three times, he then reverts to a) for several breaths. Both 2 and 3 are variants of the chest stretch. (See Chapter Six.)

4 The student stands with feet one metre (3 feet) apart, turns the right foot outwards and the left foot inwards, and raises the arms sideways to shoulder level on breathing in. Then he exhales, transferring the weight to the right hip, bending the trunk laterally to the right, and running the right hand down the outer side of the right leg, while letting the left arm rise until it points towards the ceiling. He inspires on returning to the initial position with hands at shoulder level, then exhales once more on returning to the actual starting position. The whole procedure is then repeated on the other side. (A modification of the Triangle Pose, for full details of which see Chapter Seven.) This should be performed twice on either side, then the student reverts once again to a) for several relaxed breaths.

5 The student stands with the feet about 120mm (6″) apart, loosens the ankles separately with a little rotation, bends and stretches the knees a few times—a kind of limbering up—then on a full expiration he crouches right down, placing his hands on the floor inside the knees, keeping the heels on the floor if possible, and drooping the head. It is also possible to clasp the hands behind the back while in this position, reaching round outside the knees.

6 *Cat Pose* (see full description in Chapter Six).

7 *Dog Pose* (see full description in Chapter Seven).

8 *Pose of a Child* (see full description in Chapter Six).

9 *Action breath in a 'Towards plough' position* as in A, even in a 'modified shoulder stand' position (see description of this in Chapter Seven).

D *Traditional Pranayama*

1 Bellows breath. (See B4 page 50.) This should be performed using the abdominal muscles sharply on expiration. Ten only, followed by one smooth inhalation, which is held, then slowly exhaled. This equals one round. Four rounds should be done.

2 Alternate nostril breathing five cycles at a time for three to five minutes. (See B5b page 50.)

3 The sighing breath, with the abdomen held firm and the ribs fully expanded. The glottis is held partially closed, which gives a sighing sound on both inspiration and expiration. It is carried out as follows: after an exhalation, inhale slowly through both nostrils against a partially closed glottis, then close the glottis fully, holding with a chin lock if desired (see Appendix I). Finally exhale through both nostrils. This should be performed four or five times. This particular mode of breathing is excellent to practice whether sitting, walking, or lying down.

4 The Hissing breath. Inhalation takes place through the *mouth* with the tongue flat, and its tip pushed between the upper and lower teeth, protruding slightly, so that there is a space between the tongue and upper lip. A hissing sound is then produced on inspiration. When the lungs are full, the tongue is withdrawn, the lips closed and held together firmly. Exhalation then takes place through the nostrils. The procedure is repeated three times.

5 'Bee breath' — an exercise in concentration/meditation. The ears are closed off with the thumbs, and the pupil listens to the sound of the air entering and leaving the lungs while he closes his eyes and inhales through his nostrils.

6 Swooning breath (also a form of meditation). Close eyes, focus attention on the 'third eye', placed midway between the eyebrows, and make use of the chin lock (see Appendix I). The mind slips into meditation during either the exhalation or the post-exhalation pause.

The Complete Yoga Breath

Lying
The student lies with all his body muscles relaxed so that the feet fall outwards, and knees and hips are slightly externally rotated.

The abdomen rises on inhalation but is held quite firmly so that there is no ballooning. The ribs move out and up, and finally the shoulders rise. The pupil should note all these sensations, as they occur. In; slight pause; out; longer pause. This is carried on for three minutes.

Sitting
When upright the student's vital capacity is greater than when he is flat on his back, because the gut falls away from the diaphragm. He should inhale to the full, but with no straining. Then he should exhale until the lungs feel fully emptied, finally drawing the abdomen in towards the end of expiration.

While doing this he should be told to visualise all three parts of the lungs, although the movement is one controlled continuous one. He has to use his imagination also to visualise an inflow of energy and outflow of impurities and waste. The rate should be five complete breaths per minute—that slow, but not so slow as to produce strain. The student always has to give way to his own need, and breathe more rapidly if he feels any strain. Most people with any degree of physical handicap will not be able to breathe as slowly as this until they have had a great deal of yoga practice, and many will never get there, nor should they try to.

This breath is valuable for instant vitality, and it lifts mood—depression or irritability—like the Bellows breath. Five minutes spent on this, the Bellows, and breathing in the Dog pose, if done one after the other when tired, leaves the student 'Topped up' with fresh energy for action.

Alternative to the Full Yoga Breath for revitalising
Where the previous little sequence is not possible, the following procedure can help: stand or sit with the spine straight, hunch the shoulders and relax them several times,

then roll the head from side to side several times.

Repeat both procedures about four times, and then notice the immediate improved breathing pattern.

Hold the abdomen firm, and open the lower ribs widely. This pulls the diaphragm down, so increasing the intra-abdominal pressure. Energy is then generated from the solar plexus.

Guidance to Students

The aim of breathing exercise work is the *easy* control of breathing in each of its four stages, i.e. in, pause, out, pause, and the provision of unlimited pranic energy.

Generally sit erect and alert, concentrate on each breath — be aware of the air coming into each nostril, feel the diaphragm descend and the ribs move outwards and upwards. Visualise the air going into all three lobes of the lungs, visualise life and energy coming in and rubbish, litter, going out. Imagine oxygen dispersing all over the body nourishing and renewing, loosening tension, and clarifying the mind. Air hunger — when the tissues are starved of oxygen and the body instinctively yawns and yawns — is a very real thing.

The throat should be open, and the neck relaxed. 'Sah' is the sound on inhalation, and 'Hah' on exhalation. Be conscious of a cool sensation in the throat on breathing in.

Note in all breathing exercises the active role played by the abdominal wall — on exhalation the viscera are first pushed back, then drawn in and up on maximum expulsion. On inhalation the volume of the abdominal cavity becomes smaller, because of the resistance of the abdominal wall to the downthrust of the diaphragm.

Retention of air is aided 1 by a chin lock — with the back of the neck stretched, the chin is lowered into the sternal notch, or 2 by swallowing and then not opening the glottis but freezing the movement just at the point at which the glottis is closed, or 3 by filling the mouth with a 'ball' of air, then keeping the mouth closed and the air stationary. This may always be used if the locks are found to be uncomfortable.

Besides the postures mentioned in sequence C, the following may be tried to help in breath control: All twists, Rabbit, Hare, Caterpillar, Reclining Hero and the Fish.

The order of work is 1 correct balanced breathing, 2 postures with special attention to breathing, 3 exercises specifically for breath control. The mind should be used as the observer and promoter of the breath at the beginning, but later concentration on the breath can be used to reduce the activity in the mind. This enables postures to be held longer and with more peace.

Breathing exercises

Walking
Students sometimes ask about a breathing sequence for use when walking — or when being pushed in a wheelchair, when helper and student can practise together. All or some of the following are quite practical:

1 Breathing in naturally, and then out to the count of one, then two, rising to a count of ten.
2 Full breath involving the shoulders, with the glottis half closed, listening to the sound.
3 Bellows breath.
4 Alternate nostril breathing — depending on where one is walking!
5 Deep inspiration — then hum on exhalation.
6 Cyclic breathing — breathing uniformly in cycles. Inhale one, hold one quarter, exhale one, then add retention after exhalation: One, quarter, one, quarter. Eventually the student should reach four, four, four, four.
7 Next he proceeds to different ratios: one, four, two, four or two, four, one, four. All possible variations should be tried without ever overstraining.
8 Breathing in, pausing every two seconds — four, five, six or even more times until full inspiration is reached. This is followed by a deep controlled expiration, and the procedure repeated ten times.
9 Inhale deeply, pause, then *exhale*, pausing every two secs of exhalation, four, five, six or even more times in all. This too should be repeated ten times.

Breathing while performing Postures
This can be of two types — ordinary silent breathing in and

out through the nose; or throat breathing with the glottis very slightly closed — in which case a faint sound can be heard.

There are various factors in posture work which affect the breathing. Very audible, ragged, gasping, grunting, gusty breathing all indicate to the teacher that there is something wrong to which she should be be paying attention!

The degree of concentration on the posture can make a difference — with intense concentration there is a tendency to hold the breath. With the unfit, breath is usually short and jerky, and often the air intake — and so the oxygenation — is low. This is found particularly in spastic people who may have very little chest movement, and so have to breathe at a rapid rate to get sufficient oxygen for their needs.

The type of posture also has an effect: 'strong' postures affect breathing differently from less strenuous ones. For example, in the Floor posture breath is slower, because the body is not needing much oxygen, but in the Shoulder stand it is hard to take a large inhalation because the chest is restricted, while the diaphragm has to pull against the whole weight of the legs and the lower body — with the smaller intake, breathing becomes more rapid. In the Cobra, the abdomen is pressed hard against the ground, movement is again difficult, so breath is shorter.

The synchronisation of breath and posture adds much to the value of any posture. For this the student needs to be continually aware of the breath and the breathing.

5: Postures. I

For ease of reference the postures in the next three chapters have been grouped according to their action. (There is an occasional exception.)

A Standing or sitting postures with straight spine;
B Standing or sitting postures involving spinal flexion or extension;
C Standing postures involving lateral flexion;
D Standing, sitting, lying twists;
E Inverted postures;
F Strenuous postures;

The line drawings do not cover every movement, but sufficient movements to make every posture clear. Besides the instructions for each posture, the therapeutic effect is described also, the simplifications and modifications that can be made, what the helper needs to do, useful practical aids, and the name of the counterpose and its reference number.

The simpler postures have been included, as these are the ones most within the scope of handicapped people. If what they achieve is minimal movement in the simplest possible pose, this is still of value provided the mind is working too! English names for the postures have been used throughout — the Sanskrit names can be found in Appendix III. It is necessary to turn to Chapter Eight to find actual posture sequences worked out for various disabilities, with contraindications, if any.

Postures included in this chapter: A Standing or sitting Postures with Straight Spine
1   The Simple Erect Posture
2   Head Movements a) forward/backward
                    b) lateral flexion
                    c) right and left turns

The Reclining Hero — in which the spine is extended — is included here as it naturally follows the Hero posture. The Roll Twist is also included as it is an effective loosener and so fits the overall pattern of the chapter.

1   *The Simple Erect Posture*
   a Stand erect, feet together pointing straight forward, heels and big toes touching — *not* with the feet in a five-to-one or ten-to-two position;

   b Spread the toes out and place the weight evenly on the whole of the feet;
   c Brace the knees, pulling the kneecaps up, contract all the muscles around the hips and the back of the thighs;
   d Hold the stomach in, keep the tail tucked under and the chest *slightly* forward; stand tall with neck straight, as if

the body were suspended from a string through the top of the head;

e Let the arms hang loosely from the shoulders, palms by the side of the thighs, shoulders rotated outwards towards the front. The whole body is in an attitude of openness, of reception.

Standing this way one feels light and controlled with flexible mind. The line of gravity is passing directly through the centre of the body. If the weight of the body is thrown either backward or forward the spine is strained. Balance can be reached by rocking gently forward on to the toes, and backward on to the heels.

There is no real simplification or modification of this posture — anybody who can stand at all tries to come as near to it as is possible. The helper can stand behind supporting with the hands at waist level or under the armpits, or one helper can stand on either side, holding under the armpit and down the arm. It is worth maintaining a physically handicapped person in this position, even if a great deal of help is necessary. In the erect posture the gut falls away from the diaphragm, allowing better movement in the lower part of the lungs; the kidneys and bladder drain better; and the 'feel' of balancing is imparted. A chair can be used in front or at one side, according to which helps the most, the pupil placing the hand or hands on the back of it; the chair may need to be placed up against a wall to prevent it slipping.

2 *Simple Head Movements*

a FORWARD/BACKWARD MOVEMENT

Breathe in, then on breathing out, let the chin drop forward on to the chest; breathe in and return the head to the vertical position. Next, breathe in, and on breathing out let

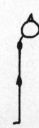

the head drop backwards, fixing the gaze on the ceiling, allowing the mouth to drop open. Repeat both twice.

b LATERAL FLEXION
Breathe in, on breathing out drop the head towards the right shoulder, but keep the face facing the front, and keep the left shoulder down. Return head to vertical position on inhalation. Repeat to the left. Repeat both twice.

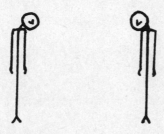

c RIGHT AND LEFT TURN
Breathe in, on breathing out *turn* the head sharply towards the right, bringing the chin over the right shoulder. Let the head drift back towards the front on inhalation. Repeat to the left. Repeat both twice.

Where movements are limited, the pupil should concentrate on breathing, leaving the moving of the head to the helper, who should work very gently, without overdoing the movements in any direction.

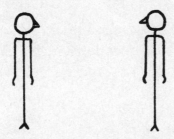

3 a Clasp the hands and place them on the back of the head just above the neck;
On exhalation push the head gently forward — if possible until the chin touches the chest. On inhalation let the head return to the starting position;

b Place the chin in the right hand, and the left hand on the back of the head. Gently move the head to the right as far as it will go and hold 15 to 30 seconds. Then let the head and hands return to the starting position;

c Change over the position of the hands and repeat **b** moving to the left.

4   *Head Roll: Standing or sitting*

Position must be erect with the spine straight and the neck and head in line with the spine.

a On exhalation slowly bend the head forward, allowing the chin to rest against the chest, then slowly roll and twist the head to the right, keeping the chin on the chest, then on the shoulder;

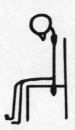

b Next slowly roll and twist the head to the extreme backward position;

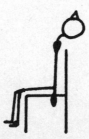
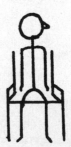

c Pause on reaching the midline at the back and inhale;
d On another exhalation start moving the head to the left, then roll the chin forward at shoulder level and finish at the centre front, bringing the head back to the upright position;
e Inhale, start exhaling and repeat the whole process, this time after dropping the head forward slowly, roll and twist the head to the left first;
f Repeat the pose from the beginning, but the second time move to the left first and the right second.

This pose relieves tension in head and neck. (Often it sounds as if little bits of gristle are giving way at the back of the neck). There is no simplification or modification and no counter-pose, nor is there any aid of value. A heavily handicapped person should be told to let the head go loose, and the helper, standing behind him, should then 'roll' the head through the movement, holding with one hand on either side of the head, finger tips pointing forward and up. Where the breathing cannot suitably be slowed, the movement should stop for each in-breath, starting again in the out breath. By getting the pupil to focus all his attention on the breath, ignoring the movement entirely, the helper may get increasing relaxation, resulting in improved movement.

5 *Eye Movements:* Sitting or standing
i a Roll the eyes as far upward as possible—hold there for one second only. Revert to the normal position;

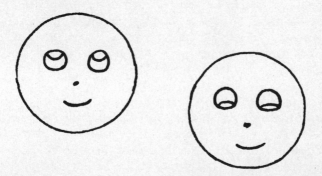

b Roll the eyes as far downwards as possible—hold for one second. Revert to the normal position;

c Roll the eyes to the extreme right—hold for one second. Revert to the normal position;

d Roll the eyes to the extreme left—hold for one second. Revert to the normal position. Repeat each movement twice.

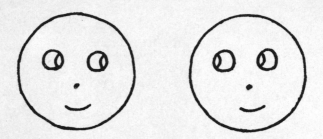

ii Roll eyes in the sequence **a)-c)-b)-d)**, that is in a circular movement without reverting to the normal position in between. Do this clockwise movement ten times.

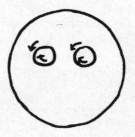

iii Repeat anti-clockwise, that is **a)-d)-b)-c)**, ten times.
The head must not move, nor the shoulder, only the eyes. A helper may be useful standing behind, to hold the head gently but firmly, fingers cupped under the chin, heel of hand on ears.

6 *Shoulder Roll*: Sitting or standing
i a On breathing in lift both the shoulders up to touch the ears;
  b On exhalation, let them drop back. Repeat twice.
ii a As above;
  b Let the shoulders down in a series of jerks, with a series of explosive out breaths. (There should be no in breaths in between.)

CHAPTER FIVE: B Standing or sitting postures with straight spine. Many of these are possible in wheelchairs.

1 Jean, Peg and Leslie working on forward bending of the head—note the neck rigidity in Leslie who has muscular dystrophy.

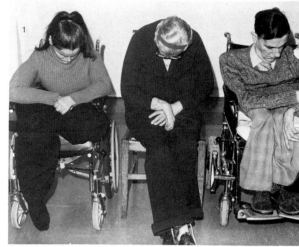

2 Bending the head back—note the even more marked neck rigidity. This is a protective spasm as muscle power is very limited and without it the head would flop helplessly.

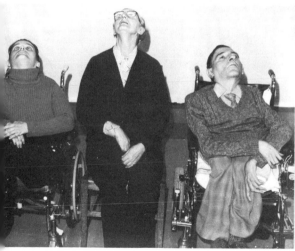

3 Lateral flexion—note the hand help necessary for Leslie.

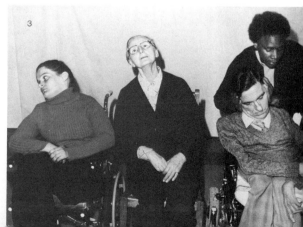

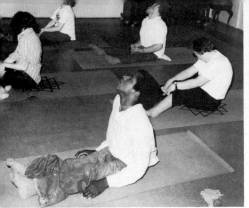

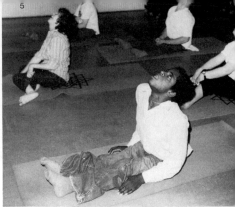

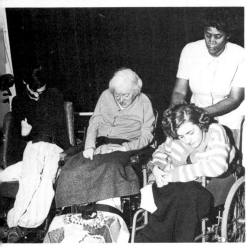

4, 5, 6 Head roll—various positions with the floor squad. Note the sitting position—Jenny, with spasticity, unable to straighten the legs, Gloria, with athetoid spasticity needing the legs flexed to the side, and the use of hands on trouser legs to keep her balanced. In both (1) and (2) notice Jenny's curved spine to prevent her falling over backwards. (3) A heavily disabled trio working on the head roll—note the helper moving the head of Denise, who has muscular dystrophy.

7 Jean and Peg working on the shoulder roll; notice Peg's paralysed right arm hanging limp; Jean is holding the wrist of her weak right arm as she raises the left shoulder.

8 Notice the helping hands with Leslie, who cannot raise his shoulders himself, and Peg's inability to raise her shoulder on the paralysed side—another helper needed!

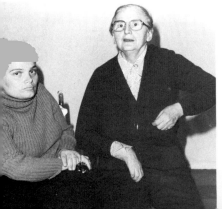

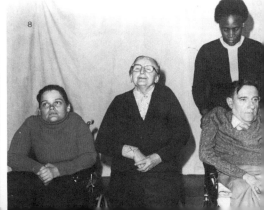

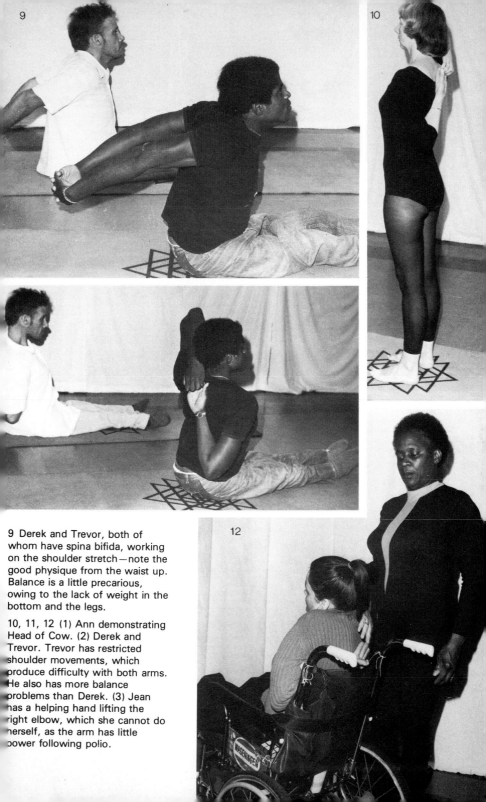

9 Derek and Trevor, both of whom have spina bifida, working on the shoulder stretch—note the good physique from the waist up. Balance is a little precarious, owing to the lack of weight in the bottom and the legs.

10, 11, 12 (1) Ann demonstrating Head of Cow. (2) Derek and Trevor. Trevor has restricted shoulder movements, which produce difficulty with both arms. He also has more balance problems than Derek. (3) Jean has a helping hand lifting the right elbow, which she cannot do herself, as the arm has little power following polio.

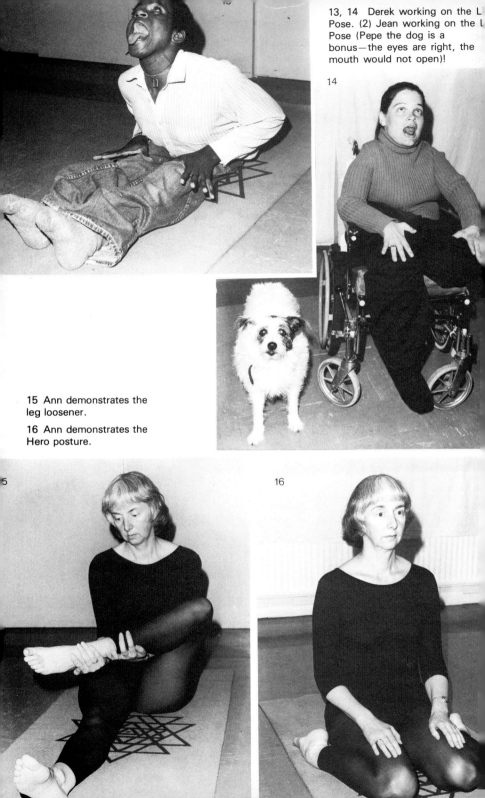

13, 14 Derek working on the Li
Pose. (2) Jean working on the Li
Pose (Pepe the dog is a
bonus—the eyes are right, the
mouth would not open)!

14

15 Ann demonstrates the
leg loosener.

16 Ann demonstrates the
Hero posture.

5

16

17

Barry, very severely
[dis]abled with athetoid
[ce]rebral palsy,
[de]monstrates his version
[of] the Reclining Hero
[po]sture. Barry is a deaf
[mu]te and learns by
[wa]tching.

Peg approaches the
[Re]clining Hero posture
[usi]ng a second chair. The
[oth]er arm being paralysed,
[sh]e can only attempt this
[pos]e.

Ann demonstrates the
[fre]e posture.

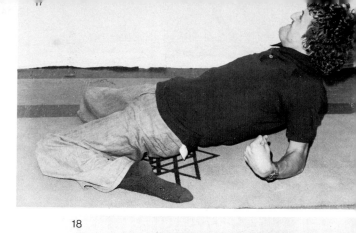

18

Sylvie, Trevor and Gloria in the
[Her]o Posture. Note Sylvie's
[par]alysed right arm, that cannot be
[rel]axed out and down by the side,
[als]o the shorter paralysed left leg.
[No]tice Trevor's bent knees, which
[can]not be strengthened when the
[bac]k (which moves in one solid
[pie]ce) is flat on the floor. Gloria
[ach]ieves the nearest to the classical
[pos]ture, but her spasticity makes it
[imp]ossible for the legs to relax
[out]wards—note the foot position.

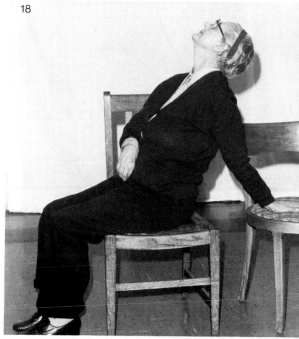

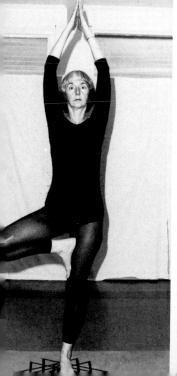

20

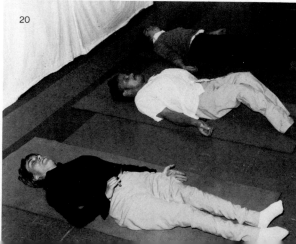

21 The same three on their faces. Note the position of Sylvie's paralysed right arm. Trevor's bottom is in the air due to the permanently bent knees and Gloria remains pigeon toed.

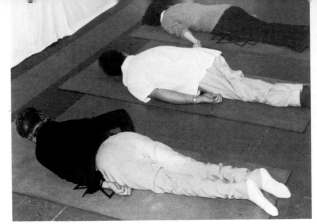

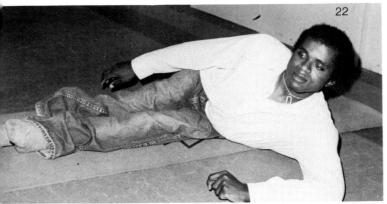

22

22 Extra 1) Derek shows one method of sitting up from lying down—throwing the weight over to the same side and pushing up on to the elbow—to be followed by attempting to straighten the arm, combined with throwing the weight forward, contracting the psoas iliacus. Sometimes it can be managed by a 'roll' of the entire trunk.

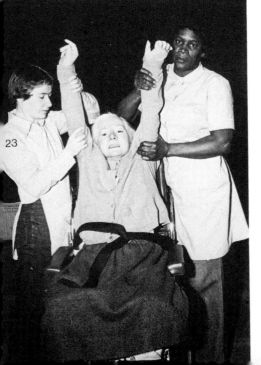

23

23 Extra 2) Working with total disability, two helpers help Doris to ventilate the lower part of the lungs, by raising the arms (See Chapter Four).

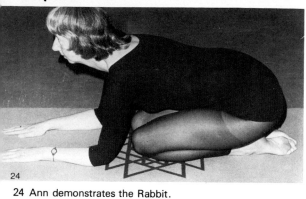

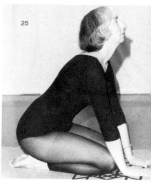

24 Ann demonstrates the Rabbit.

25 Ann demonstrates the Hare.

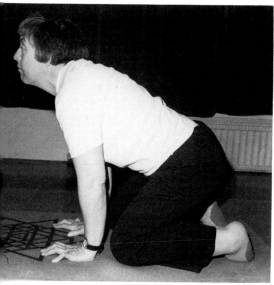

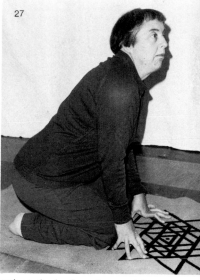

26 Jenny working on the Hare—note the inability to sit back on the heels and so straighten the back.

27 Jenny again—after a month or two she can now sit back on the heels and bring the spine more erect.

28 Massiah demonstrates the Caterpillar.

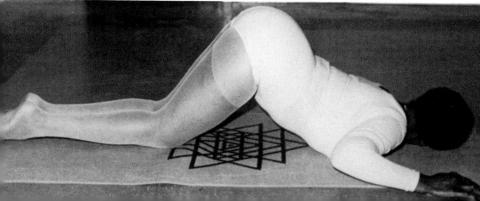

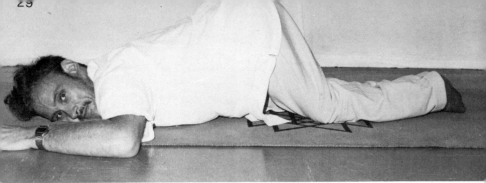

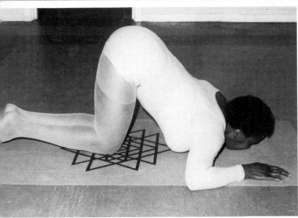

29 Trevor working on the Caterpillar

30 Massiah demonstrates the Swan

31 Ann demonstrates the Cat.

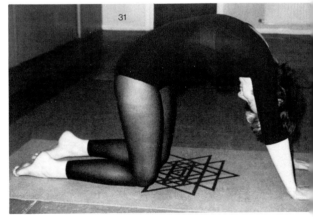

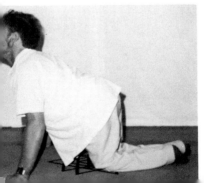

32 Trevor works on the second stage of the Cat. The balance is precarious—hence the difficulty in pushing the bottom out, note also the lack of mobility of the spine.

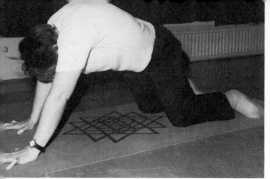

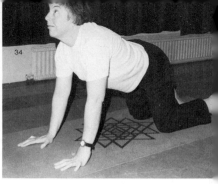

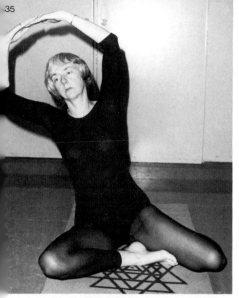

33 Jenny working on the Cat. Note the difficulty in arching the back, and the non-right angled position of arms and thighs, as she cannot yet achieve the correct ones.

34 Jenny working on the second stage of the Cat. Here the arms and thighs are better placed. Note the inability to get the feet into the correct position on the floor.

35 Ann demonstrates Spinal Flexion.

36 and 37 Ann demonstrates the standing back stretch—two different phases. (1) and (2).

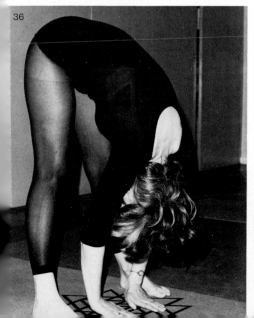

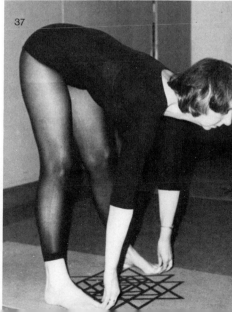

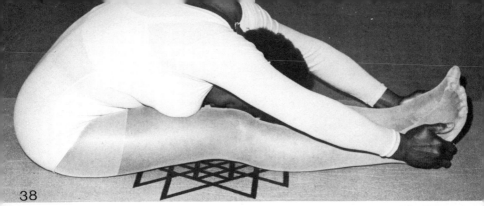

38

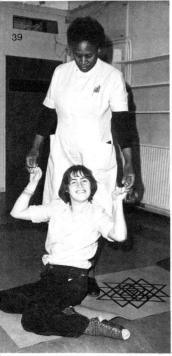

39

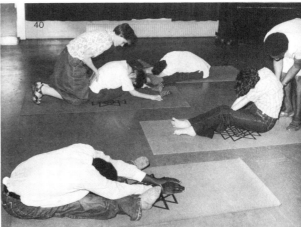

40

41 Further work on the back stretch—Gloria now has her legs a little straighter, but at the expense of the back which is rather less straight in itself, and less forward on to the thighs.

38 Massiah demonstrates the sitting back stretch.

39 Gloria is helped towards the starting position for the sitting back stretch. The helper is holding the arms until the spasms subside, before moving into the next stage.

40 Four of the floor squad working on the sitting back stretch. Notice the helpers—one applying gentle pressure low on the back, to ease the trunk forward at the hips, the other supporting Gloria who—an advance on the previous picture—is now able to work with the legs, stretched out in front—although they won't straighten

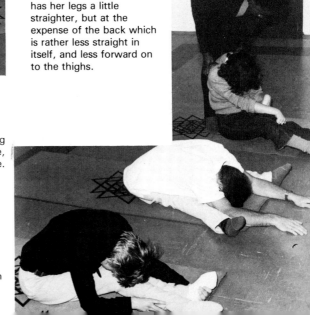

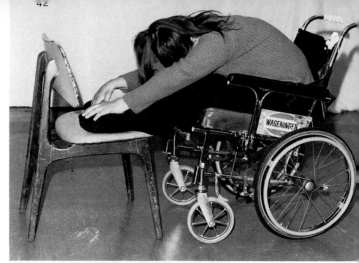

42 Jean works on the back stretch from a wheelchair, with another chair in front.

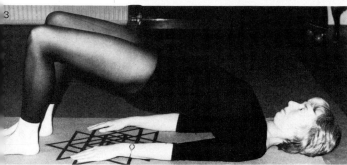

43 Ann demonstrates the Bridge posture.

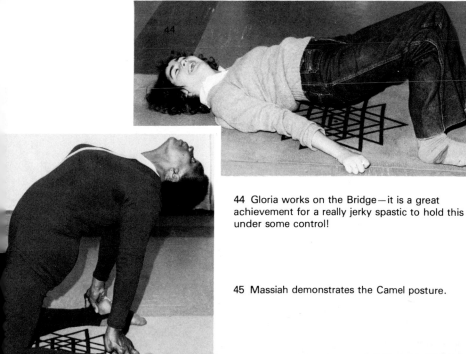

44 Gloria works on the Bridge—it is a great achievement for a really jerky spastic to hold this under some control!

45 Massiah demonstrates the Camel posture.

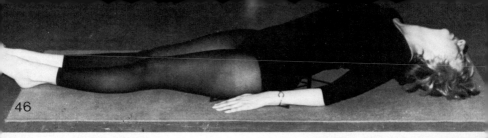

46

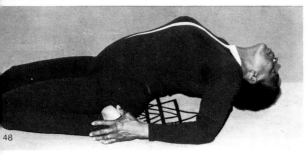

47

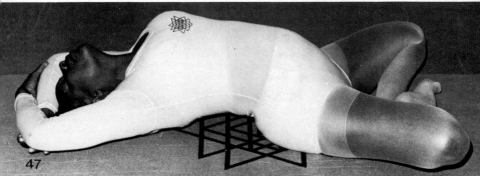

48

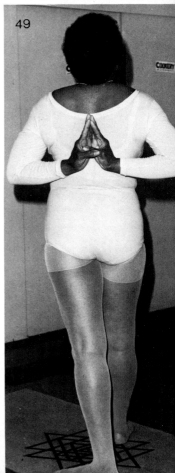

49

46, 47, 48 Ann and Massiah demonstrate various rather modified versions of the Fish, possible in some measure for the physically handicapped however severe the handicap.

49 Massiah starts the Chest Stretch.

50 Derek works on the Chest Stretch sitting down.

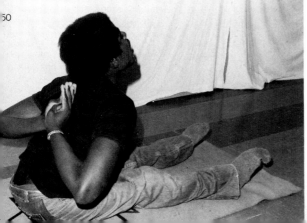

50

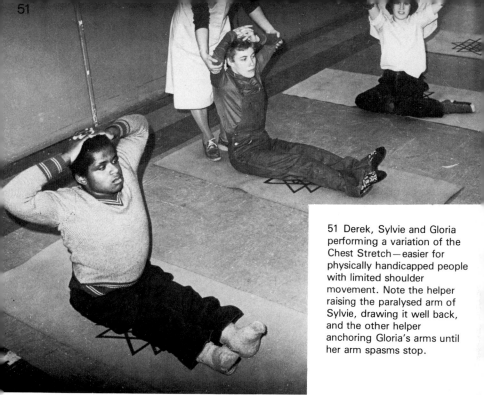

51 Derek, Sylvie and Gloria performing a variation of the Chest Stretch—easier for physically handicapped people with limited shoulder movement. Note the helper raising the paralysed arm of Sylvie, drawing it well back, and the other helper anchoring Gloria's arms until her arm spasms stop.

52 Sylvie working on the Coil. Note the careful holding of legs that will not bend at the knee, the left arm doing the work, and the paralysed right arm and hand lodged against the right leg.

53 Gloria working on the Coil. Note the way she prevents her arms flailing about in spasm by anchoring the hands under the knees. Note how supple the young spastic back is!

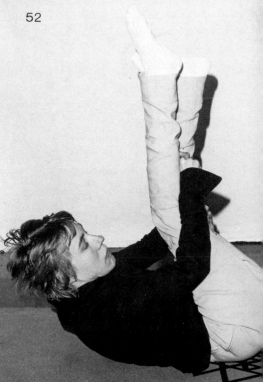

52

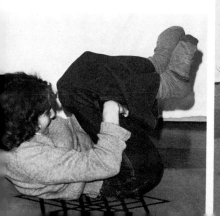

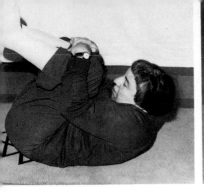
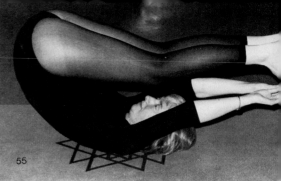

54 Jenny working on the Coil—the only one of the three who can in any way clasp her hands around the knees. Note the stiff spastic back!

55 Ann demonstrates the Slow Roll.

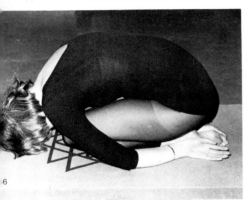
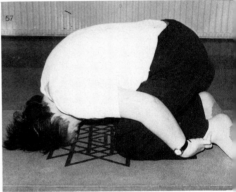

56 Ann demonstrates the Pose of a Child.

57 Jenny works on the Pose of a Child. Note the difficulty in getting the bottom down on to the heels, and the feet flat on the floor—the body just does not 'fold up' yet.

58 and **59** Leslie and Peg working on the Rag Doll. Leslie can collapse forward much better with a helper standing in front to save him from falling right out of his chair; Peg is always reluctant to let the paralysed right arm drop, but will do it if a helper helps.

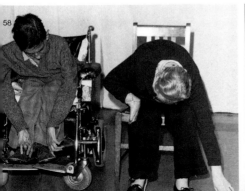
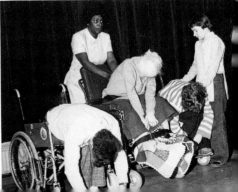

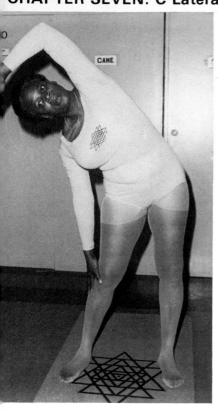

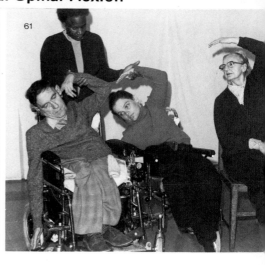

62 Gloria works on the Half Moon lying down, with the helper drawing the body into a Moon Shape.

63 Massiah demonstrates Rishi's posture.

60 Massiah demonstrates a Half Moon posture—standing.

61 Leslie, Jean and Peg working on the Half Moon—note Peg's reluctance to let the paralysed arm hang, and to drop the head (not uncommon after a stroke) and the helper holding the weak left arm of Jean—after polio, and raising the weak left arm of Leslie—weak from muscular dystrophy. Note the muscular spasm that prevents Leslie letting the head drop well over.

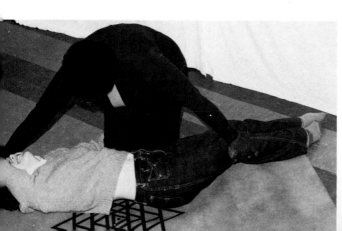

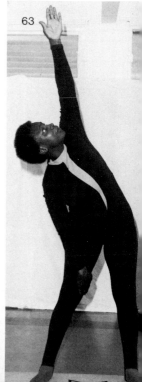

THE TWISTS

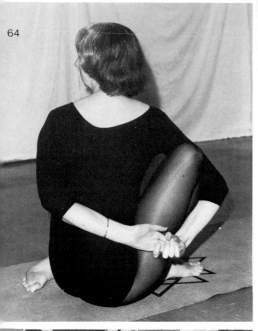

64

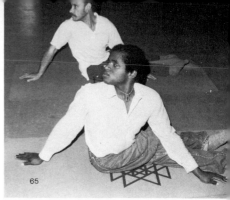

65

64 Ann demonstrates the second version of the sitting twist.

65 Derek and Trevor work on the first version of the sitting twist. Note the inability to place the crossed leg with the foot on the floor by the knee—due to the leg paralysis.

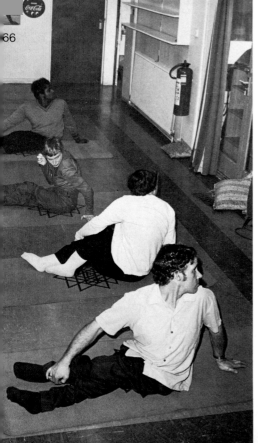

66

66 Trevor, Jenny, Sylvie and Derek working on the sitting twist. Note that Jenny cannot get her legs flat on the floor, and that her back is uniformly stiff—and slumped; Sylvie next door has the paralysed right arm in the air, and the paralysed left leg barely crossed over the right. Note the balancing difficulty she has—compare with her work on B 15) The Coil.

67 Leslie, Jean and Peg work on the sitting twist. Note the different degrees of leg crossing, their inability to get the right arm back; the helper actually twisting Leslie round.

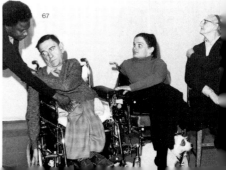

67

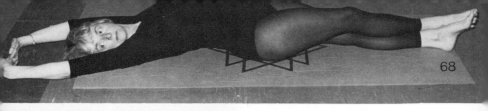

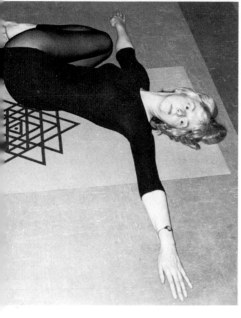

68 Ann demonstrates a spinal stretch with minimal twist, lying—all people working on the floor can achieve something of this.

69 Ann demonstrates a knee to chest twist.

70 Jenny works on the knee to chest twist—lack of mobility in the spine is very evident.

71 Massiah demonstrates the straight legs to floor twist.

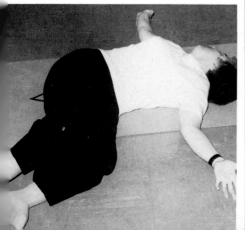

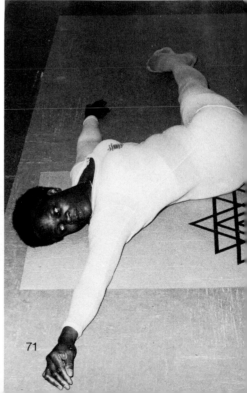

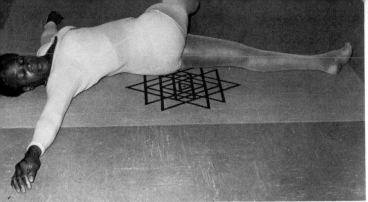

72 Massiah demonstrates the straight leg over.

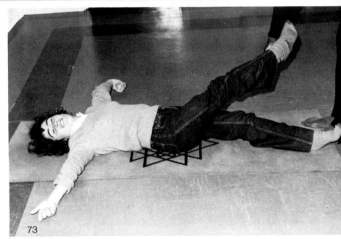

73 Gloria works on the straight leg over. The helper is holding the leg, waiting for the spasm to stop; note the helper's foot keeping the outstretched leg straight, also note the position of Gloria's outstretched left hand.

73

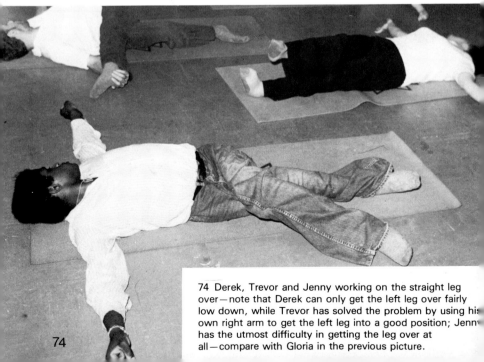

74 Derek, Trevor and Jenny working on the straight leg over—note that Derek can only get the left leg over fairly low down, while Trevor has solved the problem by using his own right arm to get the left leg into a good position; Jenny has the utmost difficulty in getting the leg over at all—compare with Gloria in the previous picture.

74

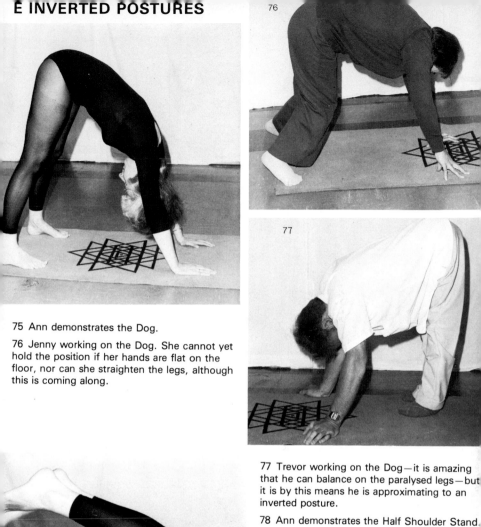

75 Ann demonstrates the Dog.

76 Jenny working on the Dog. She cannot yet hold the position if her hands are flat on the floor, nor can she straighten the legs, although this is coming along.

77 Trevor working on the Dog—it is amazing that he can balance on the paralysed legs—but it is by this means he is approximating to an inverted posture.

78 Ann demonstrates the Half Shoulder Stand.

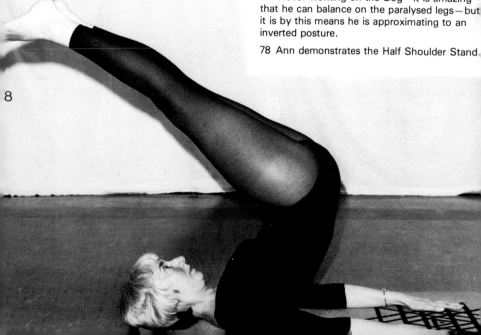

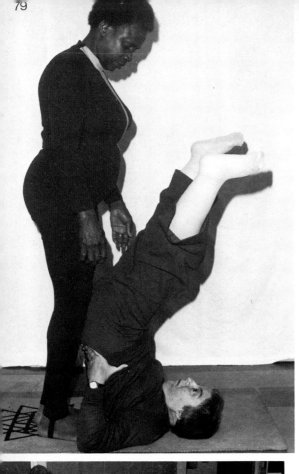

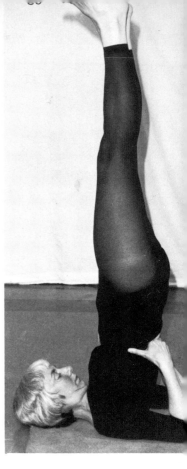

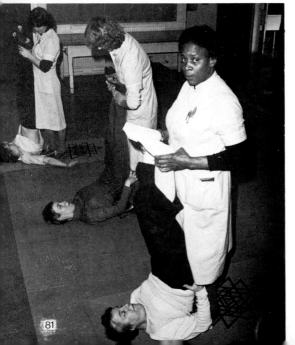

79 Jenny working on the Half Shoulder Stand—almost achieving balance. The legs, although apart, are actually closer together than they are when she stands up!

80 Ann demonstrates the Shoulder Stand.

81 Jenny, Sylvie and Gloria working on the Shoulder Stand, with help. Gloria is actually in the best position, but the helper has done most of the work, Sylvie cannot get more vertical without a helper on either side, Jenny's position is almost her own unaided effort, but she could not balance without the support of the helper's knee. She could manage without the helper's hands.

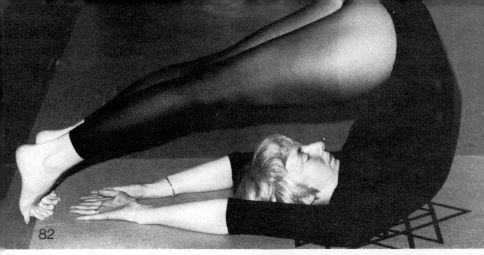

82 Ann demonstrates the Plough.

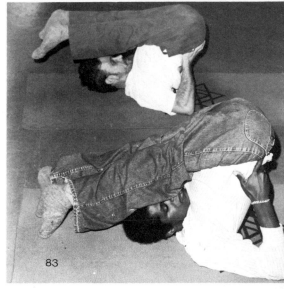

83 Derek and Trevor working on the Plough. Having paralysed legs, they go straight over into the Plough as soon as they try to invert.

84 Gloria working on the Plough. She cannot quite balance yet without the one handed support of the helper. Her own hand would be useless, due to the spasms. With the helper supporting her on either side, she can extend the legs backwards over the head quite a distance towards the floor.

85 Triumph! Jenny working on the Plough quite unsupported though — if she extends the legs any further over the head, she will overbalance.

83

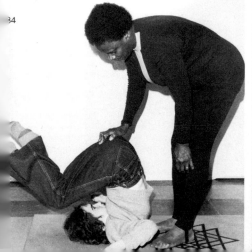

84

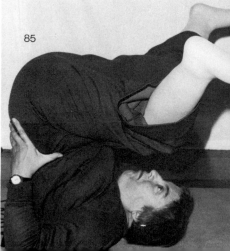

85

STRENUOUS POSTURES

86 Derek, Sylvie and Barry working on the Cobra. Note that neither Derek nor Sylvie can straighten the arms—Derek because if he does the bottom part of the body will come up off the floor, due to a rigid spina bifida back, Sylvie because one arm is paralysed, and she cannot manage on one arm alone, so rests on the forearms of both. Barry has the pelvis somewhat off the floor but this is his version of the Cobra and he sticks to it.

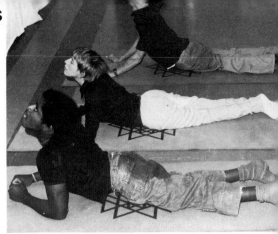

87

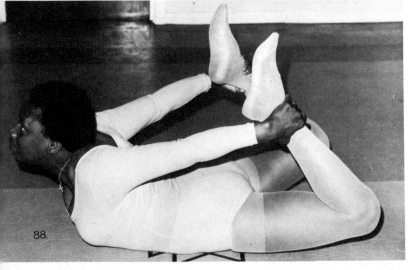

87 Julia demonstrates the Cobra. Deaf, blind and with a congenital heart lesion, Julia learns her Yoga by feel.

88 Massiah demonstrate the Bow.

88

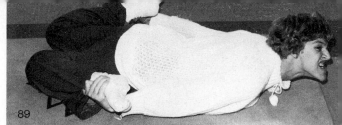

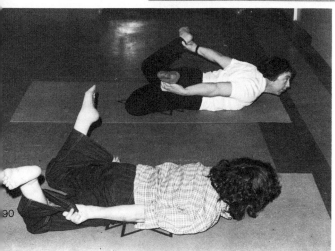

89 Karen working on the Bow. It is a great achievement for her to get her flailing arms and hands actually to hold the legs in this position. We are well content with this as a start!

90 Gloria and Jenny working on the Bow. Unlike Karen, Gloria cannot control her hand movements sufficiently to hold her legs, but manages a good grasp of the slacks. She is just beginning to get the shoulders off the floor. Jenny can lift the left leg off further than the right, but has achieved quite a good grip, and some shoulder and chest lift.

91 Massiah demonstrates the Side Leg Raise.

92 Gloria working on the Side Leg Raise. Note that she cannot raise the leg vertically, it moves forward as well. There is little support from the right hand.

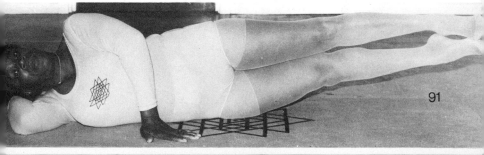

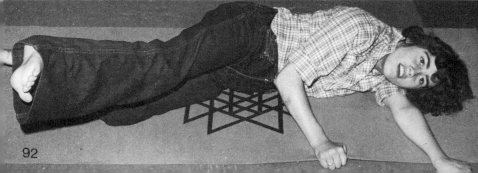

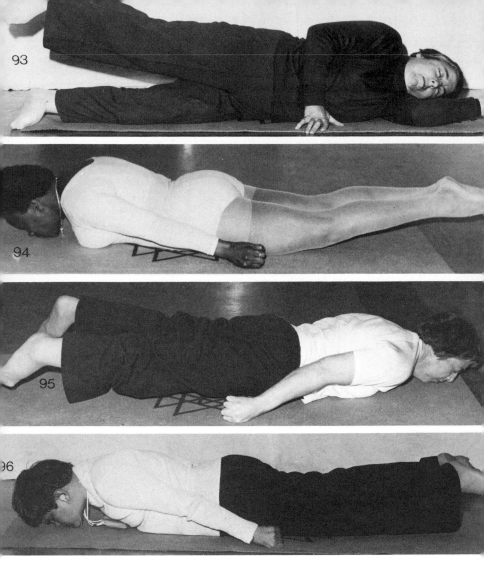

93 Jenny working on the Side Leg Raise—and very successfully too! Note the spastic right hand.

94 Massiah demonstrates the Locust.

95 Jenny working on the Locust. Note how separated the legs are.

96 Julia working on the Locust. In view of the heart lesion she is only allowed to go straight into and out of this, with no holding.

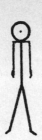 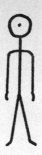

In many cases the helper will need to lift the shoulders, placing the fingers in the armpits, thumbs on the tops of the shoulders, in **1a** and **2a**. She will also need to push down in jerks in **2b**. This can be done quite forcibly to expel air from the lung bases.

iiia Lift the right shoulder to the ear, then roll it as far forward as possible. This brings the arm, flexed at the elbow if pupil is sitting, partly across the chest;

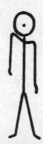

   b Drop the shoulder down as far as possible, then roll it backwards. This brings the flexed elbow towards the spine at the back;

   c Return to starting point.
      Keep the left shoulder down and the head still throughout.

   d Repeat **a)** **b)** and **c)** with the left shoulder;

   e Repeat **a)** **b) c)** and **d)** twice.

iv Carry out the movements as in **3**, only with both shoulders working together.

v Again carry out the movements as in **3**, but start with the right shoulder, then start the left shoulder moving when the right shoulder is already at **b)**. The shoulders are working rather like the pistons of a steam engine.

This whole series **3, 4,** and **5** can be repeated in the reverse direction, that is to say at **a),** after lifting the shoulder, roll it backward, not forward, then down at the back and forward in the down position.

7   *Shoulder Stretch:* Sitting or standing
   a Start from a normal sitting position in a chair, or cross-legged on the floor, or standing with the feet about 400 mm (15″) apart;

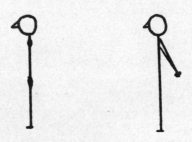

   b Clasp the hands behind the back and straighten the arms, raising them gently as high as they will go without the body bending forward, on inhalation;
   c Hold for 15 to 30 seconds;
   d Lower the arms on an exhalation and return to the starting position.

As facility with this pose advances and the arms can be lifted higher, the trunk can be bent forward, bringing the forehead over towards the floor if seated, or down between the knees if standing.

The helper may need to help the hands reach round the back so that the student can clasp them together: she may also need to help straighten the back, in the sitting position.

The Shoulder Movement and Shoulder Stretch relieve tension in that area, loosen all the muscles of the shoulder girdle and strengthen the upper muscles of the spine.

8   *Cow's Head Pose* (this can be done in a wheelchair)
   i   a If possible sit on the heels, with straight spine: otherwise sit in any comfortable position;
   b Rotate the right shoulder and arm backward, bend the elbow and place the right hand as high up the centre of the back as possible, with the palm facing outward;

c Stretch the left arm forward, raise it over the head, and bending the elbow, drop it backwards; slot the fingers of two hands firmly together, or clasp the whole hand if possible.

d Keep the head straight facing directly frontwards—the shoulders must not be hunched;

e Breathe deeply and evenly;

f Hold for 30 seconds, then release, and roll the shoulders once or twice to do away with any tension.

ii Repeat the sequence **b)** to **f)**, reversing the arms.

This posture is excellent for strengthening the muscles of respiration, because the intercostal muscles are already stretched when getting into the position—then they receive an extra stretch with each succeeding inspiration. It also loosens the shoulder girdle, and strengthens the upper muscles of the spine: latissimus dorsi, and trapezius.

The helper may need to help with the movement of both arms, including the elbow flexion, and to help draw the two hands together, applying gentle pressure at both elbow levels—one down, and one up.

A small folded scarf between the two hands may enable the posture to be held in order to attain the full benefit to the breathing.

9 *The Lion:* Sitting

a Kneel and sit back on the heels, if possible with the ankles crossed so that the right foot is under the left buttock, and the left foot is under the right buttock. If not, sit in any comfortable position;

b Rest hands on knees, keep the spine, head and arms straight;

c On exhalation spread the fingers wide apart, stretching them as much as possible; lean slightly forward, widen the eyes gazing at the tip of the nose, open the jaws widely, and push the tongue out and down towards the chin with force;

d Hold for 30 seconds;

e Slowly withdraw the tongue, relax the eyes and the fingers;

f Repeat twice. Change the position of the feet under the buttock each time, that is, making the under foot the upper one.

Children love this pose. It can be done sitting in a chair, when the position of the legs does not change. No help is needed. There is no counterpose.

It is said that this helps stammerers, it tones up the muscles of face and jaw.

10 *Finger Stretch:* Sitting

a Sit cross-legged, back on the heels, or in any comfortable position with a straight spine;

b Grasp first the thumb, then the fingers of the right hand with the thumb and first finger of the left hand, and pull each one gently three times;

c Change hands over, and perform identical movements.

This pose dispels finger stiffness, and helps to develop co-ordination of the two hands.

The helper helps where there is hand weakness or tremor, or fixed fingers, coordinating the movement, and pulling gently.

11 *Leg loosener:* Sitting

a Sit with the legs outstretched;

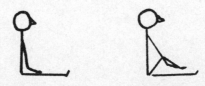

b Bend the right leg, and hold the foot or ankle underneath with the right hand, or both hands;

c Raise and lower the right leg in the air, ten times;

d Draw the foot in towards the groin, and push it outwards ten times;

e Change over legs

The second hand may be used each time to support the body. This pose loosens both hip and knee joints, and strengthens the thigh muscles. The helper may need to carry out the leg movement, or may need to support the back with the lower part of her leg, standing behind the student.

12 *Toe and ankle loosener:* Sitting

a Sit comfortably, then lift the right leg, putting the right arm underneath the right shin;

b Hold the right toes in the left hand, and rotate the foot at the ankle, about ten times clockwise and ten times anticlockwise;

c Repeat with the other foot;

d Slide the right arm down the leg and hold the right ankle: rotate each toe of the right foot, with the fingers of the left hand;

e Change over legs and repeat **a) b) c) d)**;

f Hold the right leg with both hands just above the ankle, shake the ankle and foot vigorously. If necessary use the left hand on the floor to support the body, and shake with one hand only;

g Change over legs

This pose loosens both ankle and foot muscles, and forms a useful preliminary to sitting in a cross-legged position, the Cobbler, and Hero poses.

Where the ankles are very stiff, the helper may need to grasp the foot with one hand and actually to carry out the rotation for the pupil.

She may also need to stand behind the pupil, supporting his back with the lower part of her leg.

13 *Hero:* Kneeling

a Kneel on the floor, knees together, feet somewhat apart, with the toes turned in, and the heels out;

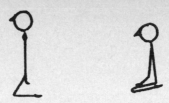

b Slowly lower the buttocks on to the ground between the calves, on exhalation.

c Breathe deeply and evenly. Keep the back straight; the outer side of the thigh and the inner side of the calf touch;

d Hold for 30 to 60 seconds;

e Return to starting position;

f Repeat twice.

Variation Interlock the fingers, stretch the arms straight up over the head, turning the wrists so that the palms are uppermost;

Hold for 30 to 60 seconds, breathing deeply;

Exhale, bring the arms down, place the hands on the soles of the feet, bending forwards and resting the chin on the knees. Hold for 30 to 60 seconds, then return to the starting point. (See B 19, page 95.)

This pose loosens knee and hip joints, strengthening thigh muscles, and stretching muscles round knees, feet and ankles. It is said to restore dropped arches. This pose can also be performed with the knees wide apart, like a frog squats. This has an even stronger effect upon hip and knee muscles.

Aid Place several cushions underneath the buttocks, and remove them one by one as tendons lengthen on frequent repetition.

14 *The Reclining Hero*

a Kneel, sitting back as in A 13, with straight spine. Establish rhythmical breathing;

b Clasp the right ankle with the right hand, and the left

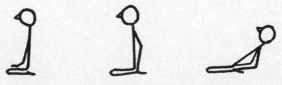

ankle with the left hand, or place the palms on the soles
of the feet;

c On exhalation lower the right elbow to the floor, rolling
slightly over to the right to do this;

d Also on an exhalation lower the left elbow to the floor;

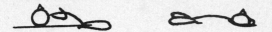

e Throw the head back till it rests on the floor, release the
ankles and join hands in prayer position in front of the
chest;

f Breathe deeply and evenly;

g Lower the arch of the back on to the floor, clasp each
elbow with one hand and take the folded arms over the
head, placing them flat on the floor. Continue breathing
evenly. Hold for one to three minutes;

(g may be omitted. It puts the posture into the strenuous
category.)

h If g has been performed, release the elbows, clasp the
ankles and on exhalation push off from the left elbow,
rolling slightly towards the right, then continue by
pushing off with the right elbow to get to the original
position. (By this means, any strain on the lower back is
avoided.)

i Go straight into the counterpose, bringing the forehead
over towards the floor, keep the buttocks on the floor between the heels if possible, the hands may be placed on
the soles of the feet.

Aid—cushions as in A 13.

Besides loosening the knee and hip joints as in A 13, this
pose extends the dorsal region, expanding the chest, stretching
the trachea, and improving the breathing power. It stimulates
the thyroid and parathyroid glands, and makes the pelvic
joints more flexible.

The helper may have to help the hands to find the ankles,
and then to support the back on the way down, placing a hand
on the small of the back, and supporting the arm at the elbow,
first on the right side and then on the left. Help is particularly
necessary on the way up, assisting the push off on either side
with gentle support: possibly a push in the small of the back.

15 *The Roll Twist:* Standing, sitting on the floor or in a chair.

  a If standing, stand with the feet about 400 mm (15″) apart: place the hands on the hips;

  b On exhalation, make circles with the trunk, rolling forwards, to the right, backwards, to the left and then forwards again;

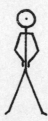 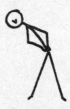

  c Return to the upright position;

  d Repeat, rolling forwards and to the left first;

  e Repeat **a) b) c) d)** twice, varying the movement from a few inches to a wide circle;

This pose releases tension, teaches balance, and strengthens the muscles of back and abdomen.

The helper can help to widen the movement in a wheelchair pupil. If possible the side arms should be removed from the wheelchair.

16 *The Tree:* standing

i **a** Stand in the erect posture. It is best to focus the eyes on the floor about 1250 mm (4 feet) in front;

  b Shift the body weight on to the left foot, spreading the toes to help with balance;

  c Bend the right leg at the knee, and using the hands, place the heel on the opposite thigh, as high as possible, with the heel resting firmly on the thigh and the toes pointing downwards. The right knee must be pointing to the side;

  d Join the palms of the hands together and raise the arms straight up over the head, breathing in;

  e Hold for 60 seconds, breathing normally;

  f Return to the starting position on an exhalation.

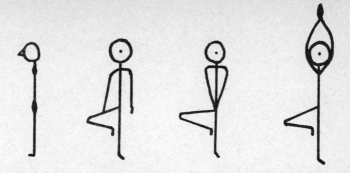

ii   Repeat **a) b) c) d)**, flexing the left leg and putting the weight on to the right leg.

This pose teaches balance, and strengthens the feet through the gripping of the toes. The lateral positioning of the right knee is of much greater importance than the height reached on the left thigh with the right foot. (It helps to press hard with the toes into the opposite leg). The two important factors of balance and external rotation of the hip can be acquired if the foot is placed *anywhere* on the opposite leg, even just above the ankle. Where necessary use a wall (or chair) at the side to give support if balance is bad, and raise only one arm above the head. After a few weeks the wall (or chair) can be dispensed with.

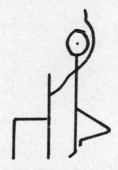

A helper may be used to help with balance or arm raising.

17   *Abdominal contraction* standing or sitting
   If standing, stand with the feet about 400 mm (15″) apart, the knees turned out and slightly bent, the hands at the top

of the thighs, with the fingers towards the inner aspect and cupped.

a Contract the stomach muscles, pulling the stomach well in, then let it relax. Repeat twice;

b On an exhalation, pull the abdominal muscles in, then snap them out with a forcible positive movement;

c Exhale fully and then repeat the pull in and snap out, as many times as possible before taking in another breath. Count the number of times. Repeat c) twice.

18   *The Floor Pose:* Lying on the back

a Lie flat on the rug with the head in a straight line with the spine. The buttocks should rest evenly on the floor;

b Pull the shoulders well down, so that both shoulder blades lie evenly on the floor;

c Place the arms slightly away from the body, palms uppermost, with the thumbs and little fingers touching;

d The feet should be a little apart, with the legs slightly externally rotated at the hips: let the knees and the feet fall outwards. The whole of the spine should be touching the floor — see below;

e Relax the jaw, have the lips lightly touching, the eyes closed, eyeballs 'looking' towards the tip of the nose;

f Deliberately relax all muscles in turn — starting at the feet (see Relaxation — Chapter Three).

MODIFICATION AND AIDS

The knees can be bent, with or without a pillow placed underneath. This helps to bring the lower part of the back in contact with the floor.

Placing a low stool underneath the legs has a similar effect. Putting a small cushion in the small of the back is comforting, but does not have such a good effect, as it perpetuates the excessive spinal arch, which has made the cushion necessary in the first place.

This is the position in which to start becoming aware, to observe the breathing (see Chapter Three).

Finally, in this position consciousness can be centred in the brow centre, the third eye — in the middle of the forehead between the eyes (see Chapter Ten, also Appendix I).

19 *The Floor Pose:* Lying on the front
   a The head is turned to one side, with the cheek touching the floor;

   b The arms are held slightly away from the body, palms facing the ceiling, elbows rolled outward, thumb and first finger of each hand touching;
   c The legs are rolled outwards at knee and ankle, feet turned in, with the toes turned towards each other.

This position is often tolerated by people who find the Floor Pose on their back uncomfortable.

Far from being easy, the Floor Pose on the back is very difficult. It is also of immense value. If attention is paid to detail the pupil has mastered the first step in the art of relaxation.

The next step is the direction of the energy flow. The pupil should become aware of a flow of energy moving up the back of the head, over the head and down the nose, down the body to the toes and back up the spine to the crown of the head.

A further step is the control of the breath. Use should be made of the breathing of relaxation (see Chapter Four), and at the same time the mind should be directed downwards towards the sources of energy within. This is easy during expiration, more difficult in inspiration: the use of a Mantra helps (see Chapter Ten).

One of the interesting effects of this pose, if held for some time, and one which shows that it has been correctly performed, is a feeling that the skin has shrunk, and the limbs elongated, coupled with a general feeling of weight, of being part of the floor.

All the work outlined in this chapter is a preparation for the more real and complete poses that are to follow, in the next two chapters. But two or three of these nineteen poses would probably be included in any sequence and even more where the pupils are markedly unfit.

6: Postures. II

The twenty postures in this chapter all involve flexion or extension of the spine, and are rather more demanding than the postures of Chapter Five, although still basic and simple. They are:

1. Rabbit
2. Hare
3. Caterpillar
4. Swan
5. Cat
6. Spine Flexion
7. Archer
8. Back Stretch (i) Standing
    (ii) Sitting
    (iii) Dynamic Versions
9. Beam
10. Bridge
11. Camel
12. Fish
13. Platform
14. Chest Stretch
15. Coil
16. Slow Roll
17. Woodlouse
18. Cobbler
19. Pose of a Child
20. Rag Doll

B Standing or Sitting Postures Including Spinal Flexion or Extension

1 *Rabbit:* Sitting on the heels
   a Kneel down and sit on the heels with the knees together, and the top of the foot on the floor;

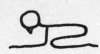

b Lean forward and place the elbows close to the knees, with the forearms resting on the floor just in front of the knees, palms down;

c Press the head back, looking up at the ceiling — squeezing the back of the neck;

d Breathe evenly and deeply.

This posture is only possible for people who can kneel, it has no real modifications. No help is required.

2 *Hare:* Sitting on the heels

  a Kneel down as in the Rabbit;

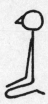 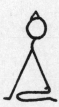

b Bring the hands, palms down, close in front of the knees, straighten up the spine as the arms straighten;

c,d Press the head back and breathe evenly as in the Rabbit.

3 *Caterpillar:* Lying

(i)a Lie face downwards on the floor, with the right side of the face to the floor;

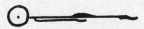 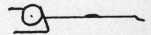

b Extend the arms at right angles at shoulder level, then bend the elbows at right angles as well, keeping forearms and hands on the floor;

c Turn the toes under, and walk them in the direction of
the head, so that the buttocks lift off the ground. The
knees, the shoulders and the upper chest are pressed to
the ground;

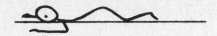

d Breathe deeply and evenly—balanced breaths;
e Relax back to starting position.
(ii)   Repeat b) to e) with the other cheek to the floor.

The helper may need to give assistance in getting the
buttocks into the air, and so tip the trunk forward to restrict
chest movement of the upper lobes. She stands astride, places
her hands under the pupil's hips and lifts.

These three poses, which should always be performed
together, begin to mobilise the spine, but their main value lies
in the effect on the lungs. In the Rabbit there is pressure from
the thighs on the middle and lower lobes of the lungs, while
the upper lobes are free. In the Hare the upper and lower
lobes are compressed, leaving the middle lobes free to expand,
while in the Caterpillar both upper and middle lobes are
compressed, and the lower lobes are free to act.

4   *Swan:* Kneeling
a Place the knees and hands on the floor, like a cat, with
the knees, shins and feet apart, and the hands directly
under the shoulders, palms of the hands and the top of
the feet on the floor;

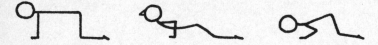

b On exhalation, bend the arms and lower the head
towards a spot on the floor, to the front of and between
the two hands;
c Allowing the trunk to move forwards, and the thighs to
straighten somewhat, bring the face down to within two
or three inches of the floor, by flexing elbows still more,
on further exhalation. Breathe evenly. Hold 20 to 30
seconds;

d Reverse all movements and return to starting point, on inhalation. Repeat twice.

This posture strengthens the wrists and arms and the chest muscles, increasing the flexibility of wrists, shoulders, hips and spine.

The helper may need to support the student into the initial position, and perhaps to support throughout — under the hips.

Aids Work with the hands on the rung of a chair, backed on to a wall, if the spine is very inflexible.

5   *Cat:* Kneeling
   a Kneel down and place the hands on the floor, under the shoulder, arms straight, so that the palms of the hands and the knees form a square. The top of the feet are against the floor;
   b On exhalation, arch the back slowly upwards, pulling the abdominal muscles in; drop the head and relax the neck muscles, but keep the arms straight. Hold for 10 — 30 seconds;

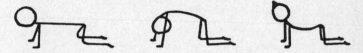

   c On inhalation raise the head and lower the back, continue till the back is arched downwards as far as possible, and the head tipped back; the bottom protrudes somewhat, but the thighs must remain perpendicular. Hold for 10 — 30 seconds;
   d on exhalation reverse **c)** and carry on into **b)** again. Perform the whole cycle — that is the pose as in **b)**, followed by **c),** five times.

This posture helps to produce a flexible spine, and tones up the abdominal muscles. It forms a useful predecessor to the more strenuous spinal exercises.

The helper may have first to lift the pupil into position and then to help lift and arch the spine — placing the hands under the abdomen at waist level. She may also need to place the feet in position — with the toes turned inwards if the feet cannot be straight. She applies slight downward pressure on the middle of the spine in **c)**, while still supporting if necessary.

6 *Spinal Flexion*

(i)a Kneel upright, on inhalation stretch the arms over the head, and lean slightly back, turning the palms to face the front, thumbs linked;

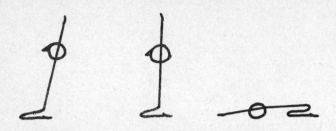

b Return to the upright position on a small exhalation;

c Completing the exhalation, lean forward and downwards, sinking back on to the heels. Slide the hands forwards along the floor until the top of the head rests on the floor. Breathe evenly, then return to starting position on an inhalation;

d Alternatively move up into the Cat position and perform as in 5), then reverse to the starting position. Inhale on moving into the Cat position and on moving back to the starting position from the Cat;

(ii) a (This pose can be performed from a wheelchair, but without changing the leg position.) Sit with crossed legs; or tuck the right foot into the groin, turning the lower leg and foot of the left leg out and round so that left foot is near the left buttock. Hold the spine straight;

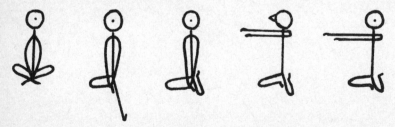

b On inhalation, raise the arms to shoulder level in front;

c On exhalation, swing the arms and trunk round to the right and hold for five seconds breathing evenly;

d On inhalation, return the arms to the front;

   e Repeat **c**) and **d**) swinging the arms and trunk to the left.
(iii) Change the legs over and repeat from **b**) to **e**).
(iv) **a** Remain seated as in **(ii)**.
   b On inhalation raise the arms over the head, joining the
      hands in a relaxed arch;

   c Stretch upwards and try to keep the spine straight; hold
      for five seconds. Breathe evenly;
   d On exhalation lower arms to sides.
(v) Change legs over and repeat **b**) **c**).
(vi) **a** and **b** as in **(iv)**.
   c Then bend the trunk sideways, keeping the arms above
      the head, and the trunk facing the front;
   d Return to the upright position, and repeat to the other
      side.
(vii) Change legs over and repeat **b**) **c**) and **d**).

This small series of poses first stretches the spine both ways,
loosens pelvic joints, relieves backstrain; second gives the spine
a lateral twist, and strengthens the muscles of the shoulders
and of the lower abdomen; and third stretches the spine
upwards, imparts slight lateral flexion, opening up the chest
cavity, and so improves respiration.

The helper may need to help paralysed or weak arms,
lifting them from underneath. She may also need to help the
trunk turn in **(ii)c** and **e**, and flex in **(vi)c** and **d**.

7 *Archer:* Sitting. (This posture is too strenuous for the unfit
or elderly.)
(i)a Sit upright with both legs outstretched;

   b On exhalation, clasp the left big toe with the left thumb and first finger, breathe in;

   c On exhalation, clasp the toes of the right foot with the right hand. Bending the knee, fold the right leg back, and lift the foot towards the right ear, drawing the right shoulder and arm back;

   d Keep the left leg straight, but relax everything else as far as possible;

   e Hold for five to ten seconds, breathing normally;

   f Return to the starting point on an exhalation, putting the right foot down, before releasing the left toe.

(ii) Repeat **b)** to **f)**, changing legs.

This posture makes the legs and hips very flexible, also the lower part of the spine. The contraction of the abdominal muscles, which is automatic, helps to relieve constipation.

The helper may need to grip firmly the hand that should be reaching the toe of the outstretched leg — providing an extension to the arm; or, where limbs are weak or paralysed, may need to lift the powerless limb into contact with the hand that is pulling it up. She can also help to draw the knee back. She may need to stand behind, supporting the spine with her lower leg.

Aids: a folded scarf round the extended foot; the support of a wall behind.

8 *Back Stretch*

(i) STANDING

   a Stand in the erect posture. Spread the feet about 400 mm (15″) apart;

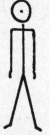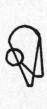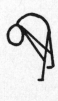

   b Bend forward and grasp the big toe of each foot with the hand, or grasp the ankles, or the legs above the ankles, keeping the knees straight;

c Keep the head up, making the back as concave as
possible — bending forward from the pelvic region;

d Brace the legs, splay the toes out to grip the floor, pull
the shoulders back; then stretch the shoulder blades,
allowing the head to move downwards. Breathe deeply
and evenly;

e On exhalation, approach the head as near to the knees as
possible — tighten the knees, flex the back, and pull on
the toes, ankles or legs, bending the arms outwards at the
elbow;

f Hold for fifteen to twenty seconds, breathing evenly;

g Inhale and return to b), then release the toes, ankles or
legs and return to the erect posture.

This posture tones the abdominal organs, activates liver and
spleen, and makes the spine flexible.

There is no need for a helper with this posture, except
perhaps to help with balance. The pupil just does what is
possible without any strain.

A counterpose such as the Camel or Fish should follow.

(ii) SITTING

a Sit on the floor with the legs stretched straight out in
front;

b Place the hands in the prayer position in front of the
chest;

  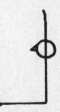

c Raise the arms straight above the head, turn the palms to
face the front;

d Lean slightly backwards, keeping the spine straight;

e Sweep forward towards the toes, moving from the hips; clasp the hands round the soles of the feet, or clasp the ankles or the legs—going just as far as is possible without strain;

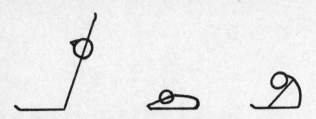

f Breathe evenly. Hold for as long as is possible;

g Reverse the movements—starting on an exhalation. Relax. Then go into a counterpose—the Camel or the Fish.

This pose can also be performed sitting in a chair with the legs extended and the feet flat on the floor; as a modification the legs can be bent—this makes the posture easier on the legs,

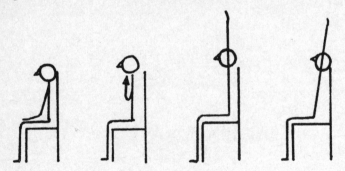

but works the back well. Putting the feet up on a low stool makes the position easier for the back. As skill increases the legs are bent less, the stool becomes lower—ie the rung of a chair.

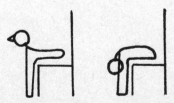

(iii) DYNAMIC VERSIONS

   a Sit with the legs wide apart. Bend the right arm at the elbow and place the forearm across the back at waist level, palm facing outwards. On inhalation raise the left arm over the head, lean slightly backwards, then on exhalation sweep forwards at the hips bringing the left hand to the outer side of the right foot. Hold for one or two minutes, then return to the starting position on an inhalation.
Change arms and repeat.

   b Lie on the back with the arms outstretched over the head. Relax. Raise the arms to a vertical position. Lower the hands to the thighs, bringing the head and shoulders off the floor, then uncurling the spine still further, move the trunk forward and down, bringing the forehead down towards the knees. Move throughout on exhalations. Hold as long as possible. If necessary the knees can be bent a little. To help in the starting movement up from the floor, the feet can be hooked under a heavy piece of furniture.

This posture stimulates the viscera, by reason of compressing the abdomen against the thighs. Both sympathetic and parasympathetic nervous systems are stimulated by the stretching of the lower part of the back, through the effect of this stretching on the plexuses in the pelvis. Mobility of the spine is developed — particularly in the lumbar region — and the spinal muscles are strengthened.

The dynamic versions particularly increase spinal mobility throughout, and strengthen the abdominal muscles, as well as producing similar effects to the static version.

The helper may need to help raise the arms, and straighten the back at the outset, and will certainly have to help in the sweeping movement forward from the hips, gently applying pressure with the palms flat at the bottom of the spine, over the sacroiliac joints.

9 *Beam Pose:* Kneeling

(i)a Kneel on the floor and stretch the right leg out in front, turning the right foot inwards. Turn the left foot and leg in slightly also, if necessary for balance;

b On exhalation lean forwards and stretch both arms along the sides of the right leg;

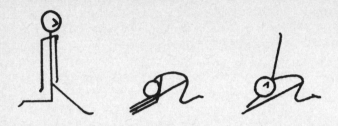

c Clasp the leg with the right hand, at the ankle if possible, or even on the back of the right foot;

d On inhalation, make a sweeping circle with the left arm, first backwards then upwards towards the head. Look up at the left hand;

e On exhalation, bring the arm back along left leg, and return to **a**);

f Repeat twice.

(ii) Change over to the left leg in front, and repeat the movements using the right arm.

This pose stretches the muscles of the spine and back, those at the side of the trunk and in the neck, loosening the muscles of the shoulder girdle. It also exercises the abdominal muscles and strengthens the muscles of the inner thigh.

Helpers may need to help to move the arms where there is weakness, to help to get the outstretched leg into position, and possibly to help the pupil to balance.

Aid: It may help to perform this posture with the side of the forward leg and the body against a wall.

10 *Bridge:* Lying

a Lie on the back on the floor;

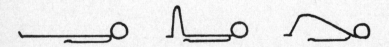

b Bend the knees and bring the feet up close to the buttocks, planting them firmly on the floor, slightly apart;

  c Keep the arms by the side, palms down;
  d Press on the floor with the foot on an inhalation, and lift
     the hips up as far as possible, allowing the chest to move
     towards the chin;
  e Balance on the feet, the shoulders and the head. Relax
     particularly the face, and breathe evenly for 30 to 60
     seconds, moving the trunk off the ground and towards
     the chin, moving higher on successive inhalations;
  f Beginning on exhalation, bring the hips back to the
     floor;
  g Finishing the exhalation, slide the feet down to extend
     the legs. Repeat **b)** to **g)** twice.

This pose expands the chest and enables breathing to be
very positive. It also strengthens the lower legs.

The helper may need to support the bridge in the middle
with a hand under the small of the back, or, for the very weak,
help in the actual lifting by standing astride with one hand at
waist level either side. She may have to stop the feet from
slipping.

11 *Camel Pose:* Sitting. (A Counterpose to forward bending
poses.)
  a Sit on the heels, with the spine straight; on inhalation,
     come up into a kneeling position, tucking the toes under,
     thighs and feet together;

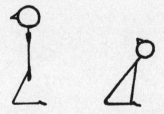

  b On an exhalation, curving the spine, lean slightly back,
     and place the right hand on the right foot, or ankle, then
     place the left hand on the left foot or ankle.
  c On an inhalation, push the hips forward, and stretch the
     head and shoulders back, arching the trunk, looking at

the ceiling. Contract the buttocks, and stretch the thoracic spine and neck as much as possible;

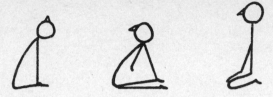

d Breathe deeply and evenly for about 10 to 30 seconds;

e Relax the arch, and bring the head to its normal position. Next, release the left hand, rolling the body over towards the right, then push off with the right hand and pull the trunk up into the kneeling position;

f Sit back on the heels.

Repeat once.

This pose compresses the spine, and the muscles of the neck and the back. It strengthens the thigh muscles and relieves any back or shoulder stiffness. It benefits the excretory and digestive systems, relieving constipation.

The helper is needed to guide the pupil's hands towards the feet — more particularly the second. She may also need to put a supporting hand or hands on the back just above the waist, if the pupil feels insecure. Help is particularly important in undoing the posture, to prevent any possible back strain — helping first the roll to the right and then the final push off.

12 *Fish Pose* — already modified: Sitting. (Counterpose to forward bends, shoulder stand and plough.)

(i)a Sit with legs outstretched. Later the pose can be done with the legs crossed, or from the Hero position;

b On exhalation, arch the back, lifting the neck and the chest, then put the right elbow on the floor, rolling slightly over to the right;

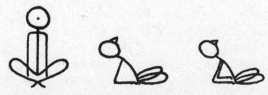

c Rolling over to the left, put the left elbow on the floor;__
d Drop further back, resting the crown of the head on the floor;
e Bend the arms across the chest, holding one elbow with each hand. Then raise arms and rest the forearms on the floor behind the head, working on an inhalation. This may be too difficult, and can be omitted;

f Breathe deeply and evenly. Hold for 30 to 60 seconds at first, then longer;
g Return the arms to the sides and push off from the floor: off the left side first, rolling slightly over to the right side, returning to a sitting position.

(ii) Repeat **b)** to **g)** with the legs crossed the other way, if the pose has been performed with crossed legs.

Further modification—just lie on the back with the arms stretched straight out over head, and the back as arched as possible. Roll on to the elbow, first on one side then on the other to come up.

Follow the pose with the forward bend or the plough, unless it is already being performed as the counterpose to one or other of these.

This posture improves breathing power because of the stretch to the trachea and the extra chest expansion. It stimulates both the thyroid and the parathyroid glands—because the neck is stretched. Also it increases the suppleness of hip and pelvic joints if performed with legs crossed or from sitting back on the heels, and corrects round shoulders.

The helper may need to support the back as the pupil gets into position, and will almost certainly need to help with similar support coming out of the posture, on both sides, in order to prevent strain on the lower back. The hands should be placed just above the sacrum to give a gentle push. Or standing astride facing the head, the helper may draw the trunk forwards with the hands in the small of the back.

13 *Platform:* Lying
   a Sit on the floor with the legs outstretched;

b Place the palms of the hands on the floor just behind the hips, with the fingers pointing towards the feet;

c Bend the knees slightly so as to get both the soles and heels of the feet on the floor;

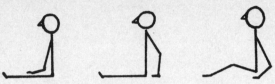

d On exhalation, take the weight of the body on the hands and feet, lifting it off the floor, straightening both arms and legs;

e Brace the elbows and the knees, stretch the neck, and throw the head back. Hold for 30 to 60 seconds, breathing evenly;

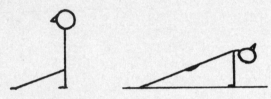

f On an exhalation bend the elbows and the knees, lowering the body to sit on the floor. Repeat twice.

This posture strengthens the wrists and the ankles, loosens the muscles of the shoulder girdle and expands the chest. It is a good counterpose to the forward bends.

The helper may have to help in the lift, placing at waist level the hands on either side; or she may keep the hands under the back as a support.

14 *Chest Stretch:* Standing

(i)a Stand in the erect position. Inhale, stretch the trunk upwards;

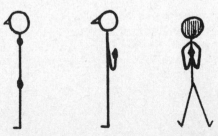

b Join the palms together behind the back, drawing the shoulders and the elbows back;

c Exhale, turn the wrists, bringing both palms together up to the middle of the back, to the level of the shoulder blades. Keep the shoulders and the elbows well back (this is the Indian gesture of respect);

d Inhale and jump (or step) so that the feet are 750 – 1000 mm (2½ to 3 feet) apart, then exhale;

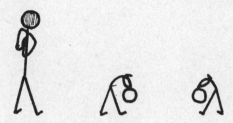

e On a further inhalation turn the whole of the trunk to the right, at the same time turning the feet in the same direction. Throw the head back and pull the shoulders back;

f On an exhalation, bend the trunk forward, bringing the head as near to the right knee as possible. Hold for 20 to 30 seconds, breathing evenly. Keep both legs braced;

g On an inhalation, slowly swing the head and the trunk towards the left knee. At the same time turn both feet to the left, then raise the head and the trunk as far back as possible as in **c**);

h On an exhalation, bend the trunk forward, bringing the head as close to the left knee as possible;

i Hold for 20 to 30 seconds breathing normally, then on an inhalation swing the head and trunk to the centre, turn the feet to face forward, and raise the trunk up to the upright position;

j Return to the erect pose with a jump or a step. Relax.

(ii) Repeat the whole proceeding, turning to the left first.

This posture relieves stiffness in the legs and hip muscles, making them flexible. The abdominal organs are constricted; this squeezes the blood out of them, and fresh blood passes in on coming out of the posture. It also corrects drooping shoulders and hollow chest. It is excellent for breathing, because the intercostal muscles are already widely separated in the initial stages, and must of necessity move even more as the posture proceeds.

The helper may need to help position the hands, and to help with the balance; beyond this the pupil should be left to achieve just what he can.

A modification of this posture is first to place the right leg forward at an angle of about 45 to 60 degrees to the body. In this case there is no swing of the trunk and head from one side to the other in the down position. The body simply returns to the upright position, and the forward leg is changed, and the posture repeated.

15 *Coil Pose:* Lying
   a Lie on the floor, spine straight, hands by the sides;
   b On exhalation bend the knees, and place the feet close to the buttocks, with the shins vertical;
   c On exhalation flex the knees on to the abdomen, keeping them together;

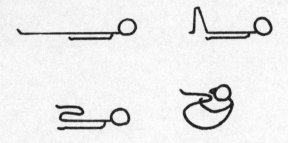

   d On final exhalation, clasp the hands around the knees, drawing the upper part of the trunk down to rest the chin on the knees;
   e Rock backward and forward on the spine, breathing evenly, 30 to 60 seconds;
   f On an inhalation revert to the starting position.

This pose stimulates the viscera and is admirable for a sluggish gut, and for someone who has a tendency to wind, or a bloated feeling in the abdomen. It promotes spinal flexibility.

The helper helps to position the hands, and may help to move the upper part of the trunk by applying gentle pressure to the mid-back, so enabling the 'rock' to take place.

16 *Slow Roll:* Lying.

  a Lie on the back on the floor, with the spine straight;

  b Flex the legs at the knee, bringing the feet towards the
buttocks — on a small exhalation;

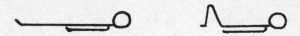

  c On further exhalation flex the thighs on to the
abdomen — as in the Coil position (15);

  d On complete exhalation, extend the legs over the head
and grasp the toes or ankles with both hands. Keep the
legs straight if possible;

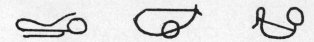

  e Rock on the upper part of the spine, three to four times,
breathing evenly, by pulling on the toes or the ankles;

  f Lower the knees towards the chin, flexing the legs, so
that the feet are just above the head, not stretched
beyond it; then rock on the middle part of the spine,
three or four times, by pulling on toes or ankles,
breathing evenly.

  g Flex the calves on to the thighs, moving the legs away
from the head, till the knees are pointing to the ceiling,
with the feet several inches off the floor. Clasp ankles
firmly;

  h Rock on the lower part of the spine — by pushing feet
down and pulling body up, moving in one piece — three
or four times, breathing evenly.

This pose massages all the vertebrae in turn, and makes the
spine more flexible.

The helper may need to help the pupil to keep balance, and
may even need to initiate the rocking movements.

17 *Woodlouse:* Sitting

  a Sit in a cross-legged position, and grip the big toe of the
right foot with the left hand, and that of the left foot with
the right hand;

b Bend forward on exhalation, and tuck the head down towards the knees, which rise off the ground;

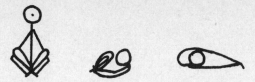

c Roll backward on to the spine, keeping the head tucked in, and the legs close to the body, pulling on the toes;
d Straighten the legs, continue rolling till the feet touch the floor behind the head, legs and arms almost straight out, legs still crossed;
e Pulling on the toes sideways and bending the knees outwards, roll back into the starting position.
Breathe evenly, timing the extreme position either way with full exhalation. Repeat five times.

This pose stimulates the circulation, loosens the spine and makes it more flexible. The abdominal organs are massaged and stimulated.

The helper needs to help the pupil keep his balance, and also helps to reach the final position either way, pressing on the knees sideways to bring the pupil into the forward position and pushing on the legs or buttocks to bring him into the backward position.

Modification Bend the knees, and clasp arms round the ankles, drop the head on to the knees and just rock backwards and forwards as far as possible, using momentum and body weight. This can then be attempted with the legs crossed, and will finally, after practice, develop into the pose complete.

18 *Cobbler:* Sitting
  a Sit on the floor, catch hold of the right foot in the right hand—fingers over the dorsum of the foot and thumb underneath, left foot with left hand similarly;

b Draw the feet in towards the buttocks, with the soles touching;
c Relax the thighs as far as possible, allowing the knees to drop down towards the floor;
d Grip the feet firmly, straighten up the spine, gaze at the tip of the nose;
e Very gently apply a little pressure from the elbows on to each thigh, in turn or both together. Hold for 60 seconds or more, breathing normally;

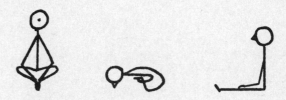

f Keeping the elbows on the thighs, on exhalation, bend forward, approaching the head to the floor as close as possible. Hold for 60 seconds or more, breathing normally. This may be omitted if too difficult;
g On inhalation bring the trunk up from the floor, loosen the hands and slide the legs straight out. Relax.

This posture is of value in urinary disorders, as it supplies blood to the pelvis and the abdomen.

It increases the flexibility of hips and knees, and overcomes the tight adductor spasm which makes it so difficult to get the knees down flat. It also increases spinal mobility.

Aid A small cushion under the buttocks, so that the pelvis is raised, makes it easier to get the knees down, and the head forward.

The helper is not necessary in this posture—except perhaps to help control the jerking movements of an athetoid spastic, pupil, holding him quietly till the movements cease before allowing him to proceed further.

19 *Pose of a Child:* Kneeling
a Kneel on the floor, then sit back on the heels, on a small exhalation;
b On further exhalation, flex the trunk down upon the thighs, keeping the buttocks in contact with the heels;

c With full exhalation, approach the forehead to the floor
   in front of the knees;

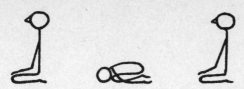

d The arms lie alongside the body, the hands being outside
   the feet, palms uppermost;
e Breathe deeply and evenly. Hold for 60 seconds;
f Sit up, back on heels.
Modification Put the fists under the forehead.
This posture may be performed with the buttocks on the
floor between the feet, which have the big toes touching and
the heels separated.
   It is a pose of complete relaxation, totally refreshing. The
abdominal muscles are contracted and breathing is pushed
into the upper lobes of the lungs. Properly performed it
loosens the muscles round the shoulder girdle.
   The helpers may have to place the feet and ease the body on
to them.
   No aids. The pupil gets as near to the posture as he can.

20 *The Rag Doll:* Wheelchair or Chair
    a Breathe in, on exhalation simply flop forward as far as
       possible at the waist;
    b Relax the head, neck and shoulders;

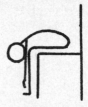

    c Let the hands hang down towards the floor, arms swing-
       ing loosely;
    d Breathe evenly. Hold for 60 seconds;
    e On an inhalation, return to the starting position.
The helper needs to stand in front, drawing the pupil

forward at the waist, holding on either side; and probably to place the arms in position in front. Standing in front she gives confidence. She is particularly important in returning the pupil to the upright position at the end, so that there is no undue strain on the lower back. She may have to support the head, for very helpless people, to prevent it falling backwards, as they return to the upright position.

7: Postures. III

The postures in this chapter cover lateral spinal flexion, spinal twists, the inverted postures, and a very few of the more strenuous postures, which in spite of being strenuous are sometimes possible for handicapped people to do. Often they are also possible for fit elderly people.
They are as follows:

C Lateral spinal flexion
1. Side stretch
2. Half Moon — standing
                         sitting
                         lying
3. Rishi's posture
4. Triangle
5. Reverse Triangle

D The Twists
1. Simple standing Twist
2. Simple sitting Twist (i)
                             (ii)
3. Spinal Stretch lying
4. Lying twist series (i)
                          (ii)
                          (iii)
                          (iv)
5. Knee chest twist
6. Straight legs to floor
7. One leg over

E Inverted Postures
1. Dog
2. Half Shoulder Stand
3. Shoulder Stand

4. Plough

F Strenuous Postures
  1. Dancer
  2. Moon
  3. Triangle
  4. Reverse Triangle
  5. Overhead Squat
  6. Cobra
  7. Bow
  8. Side Leg Raise
  9. Locust
 10. Boat

C Lateral Flexion
1 *Side Stretch*
  a Stand in the erect posture, place (or jump) the feet about 700 mm (2 feet) apart, toes facing forward;
  b Raise the arms sideways, to shoulder level, on an inhalation;

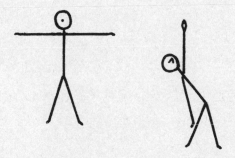

  c On an exhalation bend over sideways to the right at the waist, running the right hand down the thigh towards the knee; the left arm moving so that the hand points towards the ceiling;
  d Breathe evenly, hold for 30 to 60 seconds, looking up at the left hand;
  e Return to the starting position and repeat, bending to the left;
  f Repeat b) to e) twice.

Alternative Version
Start as in 1, but raise the arms above the head, and keep
them in this position on bending to the side.

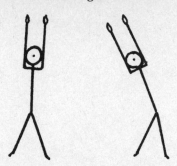

This posture helps breathing and makes the spine flexible.
The alternative version loosens the muscles of the shoulder
girdle.

This posture can also be carried out in a wheelchair — where
the alternative version is preferable.

The helper helps with balance and arm movement in the
standing version, and draws the top half of the body to the
side, helping with the arms in the sitting version.

2   *Half Moon:* Standing; Sitting; or Lying
STANDING
(i)a Stand in the erect position;
  b Place the feet about 700 mm (2 feet) apart;
  c On inhalation, raise the left arm sideways to shoulder
     level with the palm facing uppermost;

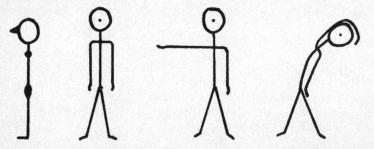

  d On exhalation bend the trunk slowly to the right from the
     waist, keeping the knees straight. Allow the right arm to

slide down the thigh, and bring the left arm up over the head, left elbow close to the left ear;

e Let the neck go limp, and the head drop towards the right shoulder; let the left arm go limp, with bent elbow, floppy wrist and limp fingers;

f Breathe gently in and out, keeping the face and the abdominal muscles relaxed. Hold for 60 seconds;

g On an inhalation, slowly revert to starting position.

(ii) Perform c) to g) using the right arm, and bending to the left.

(iii) Repeat the whole procedure twice.

This posture opens up the bases of the lungs and exercises the intercostal muscles — that is why it is so important to hold the posture for quite a time, breathing evenly and quietly. It also relaxes the muscles around the shoulder girdle.

SITTING

This posture can be done while sitting in a wheelchair; the non-moving arm hangs over the arm of the wheelchair and the body tips well over to the side too. Helpers can raise the arm, flex the elbow and make sure the arm is held well back over the top of the head, not across the face. Where the arm is too far forward the base of the lung is not opened up and the whole point of the posture is lost.

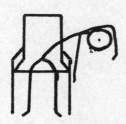 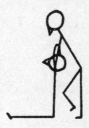

When performed sitting on the floor, the non-moving hand can rest on the thigh, or if necessary be used as a support. The helper's role is as with a wheelchair person; or it may be necessary to support the back of the pupil with the knee, with perhaps one hand under the right armpit if leaning to the right, and the other holding the left arm in position, and vice versa on leaning to the left.

LYING ON THE BACK

The movements are the same as when standing. If the pupil is largely paralysed the helper can achieve a very good posture for him by kneeling on one side, using one hand to draw the legs slightly towards herself, and the other hand to raise the opposite arm over the head, drawing the arm furthest away from her down towards herself, bringing the head with it. If the helper holds the arm at the wrist then the weight of the arm helps to open up the rib cage.

3   *Rishi's posture*
    a   Stand with the legs about 300 mm (a foot) apart;

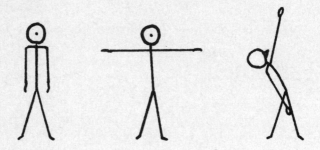

    b   Raise the arms to shoulder level on inhalation;
    c   Bend sideways to the right and slide the right arm down the inside of the left leg, to below the knee, on an exhalation;
    d   At the same time let the left arm swing upward, fingers pointing towards the ceiling. Keep the knees straight;
    e   Look up at the left hand. Hold for 30 seconds;
    f   Return to the starting point and repeat with the left arm sliding down the inside of the right leg.
        Repeat the whole proceeding twice.

This posture helps with spinal mobility, with balance, and with looseness of the shoulder girdle.

The helper helps with balance and may raise or move a non-functioning arm.

4   *The Triangle*
(i) a   Stand in the erect posture;
    b   Jump — if possible — or move to stand with feet 1 metre (3

feet) apart, inhaling deeply. Raise the arms sideways to shoulder level, palms facing downwards;

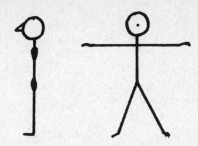

c Turn the right foot out sideways by 90° and the left foot in towards the right (the heel of the right foot should be in line with the heel of the left). Keep both knees braced and have the weight on the outer side of both feet. The body is facing the front;

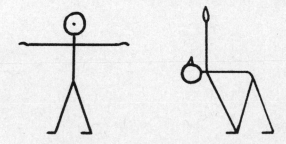

d On an exhalation, stretch the right arm, and bend the trunk sideways to the right, bringing the right palm down towards the right ankle. It can go as far as the floor, but it must not go further than is possible while still keeping the backs of the legs, the hips and chest all in one straight line. In order to do this, the right hip has to be pushed forward, the right shoulder pulled back, and the back flattened;

e Stretch the left arm up, fingers pointing up to the ceiling, and turn head to look up at outstretched hand. Pull the left shoulder back and keep the left hip forward;

f Hold the position, breathing evenly, for up to a minute. Then on an inhalation, lift the right hand from its position and return first to c) then to b).

If wanting to rest before performing the posture to the other side, drop forward at the waist, quite relaxed except for the knees—just as far as is comfortable. Let the arms and head hang loosely.

(ii)   Repeat from c) to f) turning the left foot out by 90° etc. and stretching the left arm down to the left ankle etc.

This posture strengthens the legs and ankles and removes hip or leg stiffness. It helps backache and other back problems, and develops the chest, which in a good position is well opened up.

It is of value even with minimal movement of the active arm down the legs. The position of the shoulders and hips is all important. The role of the helper is to ease the shoulders and the hips into the correct positions, and help preserve the balance. The counterpose is the reverse triangle.

5   *The Reverse Triangle*
   a Stand in the erect posture;

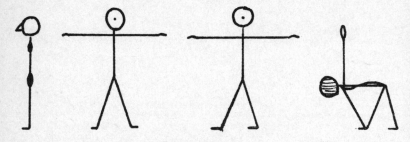

   b Inhaling deeply, jump—if possible—or move to stand with feet 1 metre (3 feet) apart and raise arms sideways to shoulder level, palms downwards;
   c Turn the right foot out sideways to 90°, and the left foot in towards the right. Keep both knees braced. The heel of the right foot should be in line with the heel of the left;
   d On an exhalation, rotate the head and trunk at the waist (and the left leg) to the right, as far as possible. The left arm is extended over the right leg;
   e Bend the trunk down sideways to the right, bringing the left hand down the outer side of the right leg towards the right ankle. It can go as far as the floor, but the most important thing again is to keep the backs of the

shoulders and the hips in a straight line, which means pushing the hips forward and drawing the shoulders back—that is, back in relation to the way the trunk is facing;

f Stretch the right arm up, fingers pointing to the ceiling, and turn the head to look at the outstretched hand. Pull the right shoulder round, and the right hip back;

g Hold the position, breathing evenly, for up to a minute. Then on an inhalation, lift the left hand from its position and return first to c) then to b).

Rest as in the Triangle, then repeat, turning to the left, reversing the arms.

This posture strengthens leg and hip muscles. It increases the blood supply to the lower part of the spine and expands the chest fully. It makes the shoulders more flexible.

For a handicapped person the rotation, even with very little flexion at the waist, is very effective.

The helper needs to help the rotation, draw the shoulders back, ease the left hip forward and the right hip back, and help to preserve the balance.

D The Twists
1 *Simple standing twist*
  a Bring the hands up in front to shoulder level, rising on to the toes;

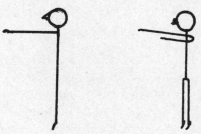

  b Slowly twist to the right on exhalation and hold for 10 seconds, then return on inhalation to the front, and sink on to the soles of the feet, but keep the arms at shoulder level;
  c Repeat b) turning to the left;
  d Lower the arms to the sides.
  e Repeat the whole procedure twice.

This posture develops spinal mobility and balance. The helper helps with balance.

2 *A Simple Spinal Twist:* Sitting
(i)a Sit on the floor, legs outstretched;

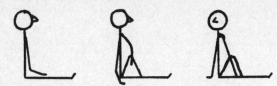

b Bend the right knee, place the right foot on the floor at the outer side of the left knee, placing the right hand on the floor on the right hand side;

c Bring the left hand over the right knee to hold left leg firmly at the knee level — fingers and thumb gripping the outer side of the knee, palm facing right;

d On an exhalation, slowly twist head and trunk as far to the right as possible, moving the right hand to the centre back, fingers pointing away from the body. Hold for 30 to 60 seconds, breathing evenly;

e Return to the front, unclasp the left hand, extend right leg and relax;

f Repeat, changing legs.

This is the simplest of the sitting twists, but very valuable. It stretches every muscle and ligament along the spinal column, increasing the blood flow. It also stimulates the nerves and ganglia along the column, the suprarenal glands and all the abdominal viscera, particularly the colon.

The helper may need to help cross the leg over, help the supporting arm round to the floor, support the spine with the lower part of her leg and rotate the head between the palms of her hands so that it faces backwards over the shoulder.

(ii) A FURTHER VERSION
    a Same starting position;
    b Bend the left knee, placing the left foot flat on the floor, shin vertical, calf and thigh touching, with the left heel close to the left buttock;
    c Stretch the left shoulder forward turning trunk to the

right, till the back of the left shoulder touches the inner side of the left knee;

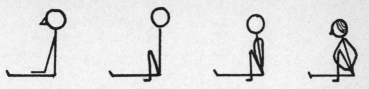

d Bend the left elbow and throw the left arm round the left knee to the back at waist level;

e On an exhalation twist the right arm behind the right side of the back, clasping the left forearm with the right hand or vice versa (or wrists). To do this, twist the trunk to the left, round the left knee: the right leg remains stretched out, the head looks over left shoulder;

f Hold for 30 to 60 seconds, breathing evenly;

g Inhale, release hands, straighten the trunk and the left leg;

h Repeat, changing legs over.

The value of this version is the same as the first: the colon is perhaps stimulated more, because of the position first of the right knee, then the left.

The helper may need to help the bent leg into position and also help the two hands to meet.

3 *The Spinal Stretch:* Lying I

a Lie flat on the back;

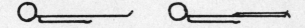

b Cross the right foot over the left, lock the two together by hooking the right toes under the left foot;

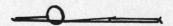

c Stretch both arms up over the head to the floor, clasp the hands together, then turn them palms uppermost;

d Stretch the arms up and the feet down. Hold for 30 seconds;

e Change the feet over and repeat.

There is only the slightest possible twist in this posture, which works chiefly by extending the spine, and strengthening the back muscles. It is included here as it is a useful start for D **4** (below).

The helper may help to position the limbs; kneeling at the feet or at the head she may gently pull on the spine to increase the stretch.

4   *The Spinal Stretch:* Lying II
(i) a Lie flat on the back, arms outstretched at shoulder level;

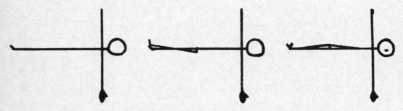

    b Lift the heel and put it on top of the right foot;
    c Turn the trunk and the legs to the right, and the head to the left, on expiration. Keep both shoulders firmly on the floor;
    d Breathe evenly. Hold for 30 to 60 seconds;
    e Return to the starting point;
    f Repeat with right foot.

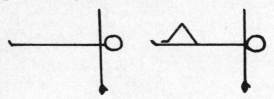

(ii) a Assume the same starting position;
    b Lift the left heel and place on top of the right shin, half way between the knee and the ankle;
    c c) d) e) f) as in **(i)**.

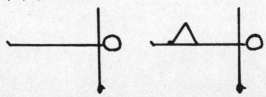

(iii)a Assume the same starting position;

   b Lift the left heel and place it on top of the right knee;

   c as in i). Take the left knee as near to the floor on the right side as possible;

   d d) e) f) as in (i).

(iv) a Assume from the same starting position;

   b Bend both knees, bringing the feet on to the floor, close to the buttocks;

   c as in (i) taking both knees as far over to the floor on the right side as possible;

   d d) e) f) as in (i).

The value of these four postures, which should always be performed as a series, lies in the promotion of spinal flexibility, the massaging and twisting effect on the spinal muscles, and the very gentle stimulation of the gut.

The helper may help to position the feet, and will almost certainly need to keep the opposite shoulder on the floor, which is vital to the efficient working of the posture.

5   *Knee to floor Roll*

   a Lie flat on the floor, raise arms to shoulder level at the side, palms to floor;

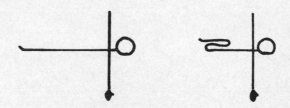

   b Flex the knees on to the abdomen, calves and thighs touching;

   c On exhalation, roll the knees over towards the floor on the right hand side — the right knee touching the floor if possible. Turn the head to the left;

   d Hold for 15 to 30 seconds, keeping both shoulders on the floor;

   e Inhale, and bring the knees back to the upright position, on the chest;

   f Return to a), repeat b) to e), moving to the left.

6   *Straight Legs to Floor*
(i) a Lie on the back on the floor, spine straight;

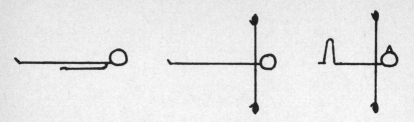

  b Inhale, stretch both arms out sideways at shoulder level, palms downwards;
  c On exhalation, raise both legs together to 90°, keeping the legs stiff and straight. If this is too difficult at first, bend knees and draw feet closer to buttocks and push off, or let one leg start slightly before the other;
  d Breathe once or twice;

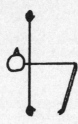

  e On exhalation, lower the two legs together sideways down to the floor on the right, until the toes of the right foot are below the right hand. Move the legs from the hips, not from the small of the back. Knees are kept braced and together. Hold for 15 to 30 seconds;
  f Keep the back and shoulders flat on the floor as far as possible, pull the abdomen to the left;
  g Slowly lift the legs, still stiff, back to the perpendicular, on exhalation. Breathe evenly for several breaths.
(ii) a Repeat, lowering the legs to the left, and pulling the abdomen to the right when in the down position;
  b After returning to the perpendicular, gently lower legs to the floor together and straight. Bend at the knee if the pull on the abdomen is too great.
This last posture stimulates liver, spleen and pancreas,

strengthens the gut throughout, and reduces fat round the abdomen, as well as increasing spinal mobility.

The helper may need to start the legs coming off the ground where the abdominal muscles are weak. She will probably need to place a hand on the shoulder on the opposite side from the legs to keep it on the floor.

7 *One Leg Over*
(i) a Lie flat on the back, spine straight;

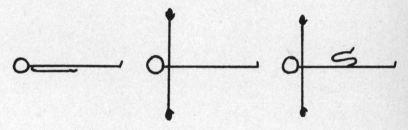

    b Inhale, stretch both arms out sideways at shoulder level, palms down;
    c On exhalation, flex the right knee on to the abdomen, straighten the leg to a perpendicular position, re-flex, and re-straighten, breathing normally;

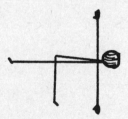

    d On exhalation, lower the leg across the body to touch the floor at waist level on the left hand side. If the toes do not reach the floor, just go as far as possible. Turn the head to look at the right hand;
    e Keep the back and shoulders flat on the floor, and pull the abdomen to the right;
    f Keep the left leg braced and straight. Breathe deeply and evenly. Hold for 30 to 60 seconds. (Legs may drop a little at each exhalation);
    g Return to the upright position on an exhalation, flex,

and re-straighten the leg, then flex and return to the outstretched position on the floor alongside the other leg.

(ii)   Repeat, changing legs.

This pose stimulates the pelvic viscera, and strengthens the muscles of the chest — pectorals and intercostals.

The helper may need to support the leg once it has come across, and help it towards waist level, before allowing it to reach the ground much lower down, towards the ankle, by means of its own weight.

She may also need to anchor the opposite shoulder.

With the whole series of twists, the helper may need to assist in the actual twisting movement. What she must *not* do is force the knees to the ground in 4 (ii), (iii), and (iv), or 5.

In 6, she may find it necessary to help the legs to return to the upright position from the floor on either side. It is very important that this movement should not strain the lower back — which will easily happen where the inner muscles working on the spine (psoas — iliacus) are weak.

Aids The pupil may hold on to the leg of a heavy chair or similar to keep the shoulder on the ground, throughout the lying twists.

E Inverted Postures

The Dog pose, which starts this section, is not, strictly speaking, an inverted posture. However many of its benefits are those of the inverted postures, and it may be the only inverted posture that it is wise for some handicapped people to attempt.

1 *Dog Pose*

    a Lie on the front on the floor, place the palms of the hands flat on the floor at shoulder level, then turn the toes under with the feet about 300 mm (1 foot) apart;

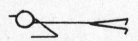 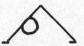

    b On an exhalation, press with the hands and push up, raising the shoulders and arching the back. Then push

backwards, bringing the bottom into the air. Straighten
the arms to form an inverted V;

c Keep the head down between the arms, and the knees
braced. Bring the heels down as close to the floor as
possible, pulling the abdomen in;

d Breathe deeply and evenly;

e Hold for 30 to 60 seconds;

f On exhalation; stretch trunk forward and lower the
body to floor. (If necessary, put the knees down first.)

This pose removes fatigue when one is exhausted,
stimulating the circulation to the brain. It overcomes stiffness
in the heels, lengthens the Achilles tendon and strengthens the
ankles. It also relieves stiffness of the shoulder joints and
strengthens the abdominal muscles, which contract automatically. The heart beat slows, the head, eyes and nasal
passages all get an extra supply of blood.

The helper may need to assist the student into this position,
lifting the trunk up and back. She may also have to prevent
the feet slipping if the toes cannot grip the floor.

Aids It may be helpful to place the hands on the seat of a
chair set against a wall, perhaps starting from a standing position if this is easier, then proceed to the rung of a chair, and
hence to the floor.

2 *The Half Shoulder Stand*

a Lie on the back on the floor, spine straight, with the
arms down by the sides, head in a straight line with the
body. Relax;

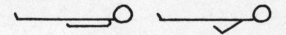

b Bend the arms slightly at the elbow, so as to be able to
apply pressure with the hands on the floor;

c On an inhalation, raise both legs 45°, or bend the knees
and draw up towards the chest, until the thighs are
pressing on the stomach;

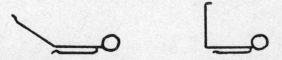

d With a slight exhalation raise the legs to 90°;

e Using hand pressure on the floor, on further exhalation, lift both legs over the head, parallel with the floor; the hands are taking a good deal of the weight. (Or if this is not possible, raise the hips from the floor using the hands on the lower back at hip level);

f Breathing in, lift both legs up towards the ceiling, but keep the body bent at the waist. The feet are kept flat. The hands are placed at the waist level of the back as a support;

g Breathe evenly. Hold for as long as is possible;

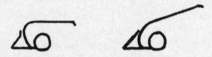

h On an exhalation, lower the legs over the head, so that they are parallel with the floor;

i Breathe evenly. Hold for 30 to 60 seconds, then revert to the position as in **f**), revert to **d**) on partial inhalation and **c**) on full inhalation;

j Lower the legs to the floor on exhalation, relax, then go into a counterpose, such as the Cobra.

For the value, the work of the helper and possible aids, see **E 3** below, the Full Shoulder Stand.

3 *The Shoulder Stand*

   a as in **2**, also **b**), **c**), **d**);

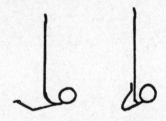

e On an exhalation, raise both legs towards the ceiling, the whole body making a line vertical to the floor, pushing down on the floor with the hands as necessary;

f Lock the chin into the sternal notch, use the hands to support the back about halfway up in the middle of the spine, with the elbows remaining on the floor, not wider

apart than the shoulders. In this posture *only* the back
of the head, the neck, the shoulders, and the backs of
the arms down to the elbows are on the floor;

g Breathe evenly, hold as long as possible. If comfortable
and proficient, use some variations; if desired, go into
the plough (see **E 4**) and return. Open the legs as a pair
of scissors, hold for a minute then change the direction
of each leg. If the legs swing out of the vertical, tighten
the back thigh muscles and stretch the legs. Keep the
elbows not further apart than the shoulders throughout;

h Release the hands, and let the back slide down on to the
floor, gently and gradually, not in one great jerk.
Relax, then go into the counterpose.

This posture is one of the most valuable of all yoga postures,
the benefits of the half posture being very similar to those of
the full. The full shoulder stand has a general toning effect on
the thyroid, whereas the half stand leaves the neck more free,
so allowing a strong flow of blood to the cervical area. Apart
from this, both postures benefit all parts of the body. Being
inverted postures, they reverse the normal pull which gravity
exercises on the organs; the blood flow to the head is
increased, so that the poses are invigorating and relieve
fatigue. The skin of the face and the hair both receive extra
oxygen from the increased blood supply, as does the chest.
Surplus blood is drained from the legs and the abdominal
organs: any dropping of the abdominal organs due to poor
muscle tone is reversed. Chest breathing is restricted because
the chin presses into the sternal notch, hence the diaphragm is
forced into greater activity. Deep abdominal breathing
results, with powerful massaging effect upon all the
abdominal organs. The pose is particularly good for eradicat-
ing pain, stiffness and tension in the neck.

The helper has a large and varied role with this pose. First
she may have to help to get the legs up off the floor, and up on
to the chest. Often help is also needed, particularly for over-
weight people, to get the bottom up off the floor — this can be
done by standing at the foot end of the body and lifting, pushing or even by pulling on the legs. Where the back is weak,
help may be required for balancing purposes, or to reach the
actual final position in both half and full shoulder stands.

Help is also often necessary to prevent the pupil coming out of the pose in a great jerk, which puts an immense strain on the bottom of the back. The helper needs to control this into a slow movement, with the back unfolding.

Aids The pupil may lie on his back and approach the bottom as near to a wall as possible. Then he lifts the legs up the wall—or a helper can do this for him—so that the wall takes the weight of the legs. With a helper raising on either side, it may be possible to take the buttocks a little off the floor.

4   *The Plough:* Lying

(i) **a** Lie on the back on the floor, spine straight, with the back as flat on the floor as possible. Relax;

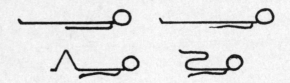

  b Bend the arms slightly at the elbows so as to be able to apply pressure to the floor with the hands;
  c On inhalation, bend the legs at the knee, bringing the feet near the buttocks;
  d On a small exhalation lift the bent knees on to the chest: feet must be relaxed. (This **c**) and **d**) may be the method used in the shoulder stand);

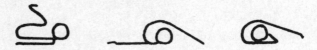

  e On further exhalation raise the legs and buttocks so that the knees rest on the forehead, with the shins vertical (be careful not to point the toes). Pressure with the hand or fingers on the floor helps into this position and takes any strain off the abdomen;
  f On complete exhalation, bring the feet and legs over the head, and the feet on to the floor, behind the head, stretching the legs as far back as possible. The arms are on the floor pointing straight down in the opposite direction to the legs;
  g Clasp the wrists, slide the hands up to the elbows, and

pull the shoulders down, thus stretching the spine
completely;

h Lock the chest against the chin;

i Relax, breathe deeply and easily. Hold as long as
possible.

(ii) *Variations*

    a Toes may be turned under, hands may be clasped below
the bottom;

    b The hands may be placed on the lower part of the back;

    c The hands and arms may be extended above the head to
clasp each other or reach the toes;

    d The knees may be flexed, and placed on the floor,
pressing on the ears—duration 30 to 60 seconds.

(iii) On coming out of the pose, reverse the movements—moving always on inhalation.

    a Lift the feet off the ground behind the head and bring
the knees on to the forehead, with the hands taking the
strain, by pressing on the floor near the bottom;

    b Unwind the back, until the legs are at 90° to the chest,
buttocks on the floor, hands and head also on the floor;

    c Lower the feet to the floor near the buttocks, then slide
the legs out straight;

    d Relax, breathe evenly. Move into the counter-
pose—Cobra, Fish, Reclining Hero.

(iv) It is useful to move into the plough from the shoulder
stand:

    a Release chin lock, and lower the trunk slightly;

    b Bring the legs over the head, with the feet touching the
floor; move the arms back until the hands touch the
outstretched feet;

    c Brace the knees by contracting thigh muscles—this
raises the trunk;

    d Support the trunk in the perpendicular position,
putting hands in the middle of the back, if desired, or
keep them as in **b)**, or stretch arms downwards beyond
the bottom.

The value of this pose is the same as the shoulder stand, with extra benefits to the abdominal organs due to compression and flushing. The spine gets an extra supply of blood because it is well stretched. The helper helps as in the shoulder stand.

Aids In the early stages a stool may be placed behind the head, or a pile of cushions, for the feet to rest on if the feet have difficulty in reaching the floor, or if the breathing is incommoded.

F Strenuous Postures

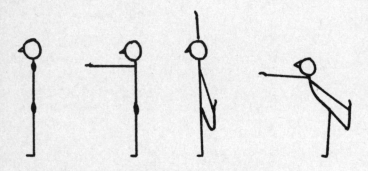

1   *The Dancer* Standing

This is not a strenuous posture if the position is not taken far out of the vertical — the greater the forward inclination of the trunk, and backward extension of the leg, the more strenuous it becomes.

a   Stand erect, feet pointing towards the front;

b   Raise the right arm in front, to shoulder level;

c   Bend the left knee, bringing the left foot up behind the knee, pull the knee cap taut and brace the leg;

d   Hold the left ankle with the left hand, at the same time raising the right arm higher, above the head;

e   On inspiration, incline the body forward, bringing the right arm lower again towards shoulder level, and extend and raise the left leg backwards;

f   Hold 30 to 60 seconds;

g   Return to starting position. Repeat, changing legs.

This posture strengthens the legs and develops balance. It strengthens the shoulder muscles and expands the chest.

The helper helps with balance, and the finding of the foot with the hand.

2   *The Moon Pose:* Standing

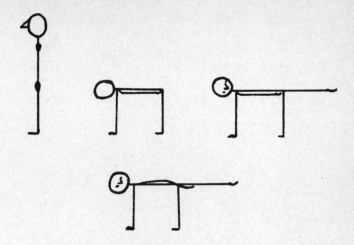

(i) a Stand in the erect posture;

    b Bend forwards at the hips and place the right hand on the floor, at a convenient distance in front — keeping the legs straight if possible;

    c Lock the right leg at the knee, and raise the left leg backwards off the floor until it is parallel to the floor at hip level;

    d Place the left hand straight down the left thigh, at the side or on the under surface as a support;

    e Turn chest to left, then turn the head to look backwards along the left leg;

    f Hold for 5 to 10 seconds, then return to the erect position.

(ii) Repeat, standing on left leg.

    Repeat the whole procedure once.

This pose strenghtens the legs, the lower part of the spine, the knees and the feet. It promotes confidence and a sense of balance.

The helper may have to help raise and support the leg, and help to preserve balance.

A useful aid is a low stool for the outstretched hand, if the spine and hips are stiff.

A further aid is the use of a chair. Stand some distance from it and hold the back, at first with outstretched arms, then reduce this to one arm, eventually turning the trunk sideways, as in **e)** above. Later, the procedure is transferred to the seat of the chair, then to the stool, finally to the floor.

3 *Triangle* See **C 4**
4 *Reverse Triangle* See **C 5**

5   *The Squat:* Standing

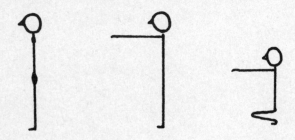

a Stand with the feet together;
b On inspiration, bring the arms up in front to shoulder level;
c On expiration, bend at the knees, keeping the back straight and the heels on the floor if possible;
d Go down just as far as is possible, hold for 30 seconds;
e On inspiration, return to the starting point. Repeat twice.

This posture strengthens the calf and thigh muscles, improves the flexibility of the knees, and promotes balance.

The helper helps with balance, and may serve as something solid for the pupil to hold on to.

Aids A table top is useful for the pupil to lean on, or he may hold on to the two handles of an opened door, or the back of a chair if this is steady enough. A book or cushion is useful under the heels.

6   *Cobra:* Lying

(i) a Lie on the face on the floor, spine straight, with the top of the feet resting on the floor, head turned to one side, resting on the cheek, arms straight down by the side of the body, relaxed;

b On an inhalation, bring the head and shoulders off the floor, arching the spine, and drawing the shoulders together at the back. Contract the buttocks and the perianal muscles;

c Breathe deeply and evenly. Hold for 15 to 30 seconds;

d Relax down on exhalation. Repeat twice.

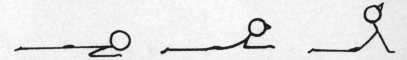

(ii) a Place the hands, palms down at shoulder level, with the fingers pointing forwards. Keep the elbows close to the sides, with the whole of the forearms on the ground;

b On an inhalation raise the head and shoulders and arch the back as in (i);

c On reaching the limit, press on the hands, and arch the back a little more, keeping the pelvis on the ground; the arms remain slightly bent;

d Tilt the head and neck back, looking upwards, but do not allow the neck to vanish between the shoulders;

e Breathe evenly and deeply, relax the back and the whole of the body except the arms. Hold for 15 to 60 seconds;

f On an exhalation gradually allow body to return to the starting position, finally turning the head to rest the other cheek on the floor;

g Repeat twice, then go into the counterpose — the back stretch, or plough — unless the Cobra was itself being performed as a counterpose.

This posture strengthens the spinal muscles from the cervical to the lumbar regions, promoting flexibility. It straightens and improves drooping shoulders or a hollow chest. All the nerves and sympathetic ganglia on both sides of the spine are stimulated, so benefitting all organs. It removes stagnant blood from the mid-back area by compression, thus stimulates an inflow of fresh oxygenated blood. The kidneys in particular are well flushed and massaged. By means of the deep breathing, intra-abdominal pressure is increased, which gently squeezes the viscera, resulting in improved functioning of the digestive system. Blood supply to the pelvic organs is also increased.

The pose also stimulates both the adrenals and the supra-renals, with profound long-term effects.

The helper may need to help the backwards flexion of the spine very gently where this is rigid, by standing astride, placing the fingers over the front of the shoulders and raising the body gently; also where paralysed or weak arms make it impossible to push the body off the floor. Spastic people, in particular any with athetoid movements, need to be helped by pressure on the legs at ankle level so as to give them something to 'work against'. This helps the arching of the back back-wards.

7   The Bow

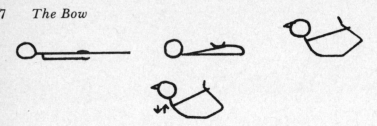

a Lie on the face with the tops of the feet on the floor, arms alongside the body, palms uppermost;

b Exhale and bend the knees, stretch the arms back and hold the left ankle with the left hand and the right ankle with the right hand. Keep the feet together, and the knees slightly apart. Keep the back relaxed;

c Inhale. Exhale. Inhale again;

d On exhalation, pull the legs up, raising the knees off the floor by contracting the calves and thighs, simultane-ously lift the chest off the floor; then join thighs, knees, ankles together, if possible;

e Breathe normally. Hold for 10 to 20 seconds, then relax into the starting position, or rock the body backwards and forwards a few times—breathing in on rocking backwards, and out on rocking forwards;

f Relax the pull on the legs, and first let one subside on to the floor, then the other. Lower the head to the floor and turn the face to one side. Relax. Then repeat once.

This posture promotes the elasticity of the spine, tones up and massages the abdominal viscera, improves digestion, relieves constipation; it enables the body to store energy, stimulating the solar plexus. It also stimulates the adrenals, suprarenals and thyroid. The muscles of chin, chest, abdomen, and thighs are all stretched. The rocking movements strongly increase the circulation.

The helper may need to assist the pupil to reach the ankle — particularly the second ankle — with the hand. She may have to hold the hand in place, acting as an extension between hand and ankle.

Aids Where the gap between hand and ankle is very great, a flat strong scarf, ends held in the hands, for the ankles to push out against, coupled with a cushion beneath the thighs, gives the 'feeling' of the posture.

8   *The Simple Side Leg Raise:* Lying

This too is not a very strenuous posture, but it is inserted here as it is useful to perform it on one side between the Cobra and the Locust and on the second side after the Locust.

   a Lie on the right side, making a straight line from head to toe, with the left hand on the floor, in front of the middle of the body as a support;
   b On breathing in, raise the left leg, hold for 10 seconds, then lower it. Repeat twice;
   c Breathing in, raise both legs — pushing on the floor with the left hand. Hold for five seconds, then relax, lowering the legs;
   d Turn over, repeating a) to c) on the other side, or perform the Locust first and then the second part of the simple side leg raise.

9   *The Locust:* Lying

   a Lie on the front, hands by the sides, the tops of the feet on the floor;
   b On an inhalation lift the right leg off the floor, as high as possible, extending the leg at the hip and thigh. The

clenched fists may be pressed into the floor to help contract the buttocks and the perianal muscles;

c   Breathe evenly and deeply. Hold for 30 seconds;

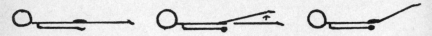

d   On an exhalation, allow the leg to return to the floor. Relax;

e   Repeat the procedure with the left leg;

f   Repeat raising both legs, keep the knees and the ankles together.

The pose aids digestion, and relieves flatulence. It massages the kidneys, and stimulates the abdominal viscera. It also makes the spine flexible, and strengthens the muscles of the lumbar spine.

The helper may need to help keep the leg straight, should it flex automatically at the knee when the pupil tries to raise it. She should insert a hand flat beneath the knee, and raise gently. Where the pupil cannot raise the leg at all himself, one hand beneath the knee and one beneath the ankle may be used.

Where the pupil is very close to being able to raise his leg but cannot quite make it, it may help if the helper pulls on it at the ankle. If the pupil places his own hands under his thighs, he may perhaps be able to push them up himself.

10   *The Boat:* Sitting

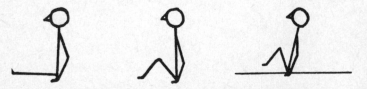

(i) a   Sit on the floor, legs outstretched, palms flat on the floor (knees may be bent and feet slightly nearer to the body, to make the pose easier in the early stages);

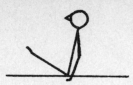

b On exhalation, lean back, raising the legs off the ground or — if starting with bent knees — raise the legs and straighten the knees. The feet should come no higher than the face. Balance, breathing evenly for a few seconds;

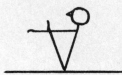 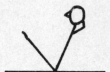

c Again on exhalation, stretch the arms on either side of the legs, keeping the back straight. The body is balanced on the buttocks;

d Be very careful not to hold the breath; breathe evenly, not deeply, hold for 10 to 20 seconds;

e On inhalation, lower the hands to the ground on either side of the hips, then the legs.

(ii)   *Variation*

The fingers may be interlocked and hands placed just behind the head, above the nape of the neck. In this variation the legs and arms move simultaneously. Strong abdominal muscles are necessary.

This pose strengthens the thigh and abdominal muscles, which contract automatically; also the muscles of the back; and stimulates liver, gall bladder, spleen.

The helper works by lifting the legs, and with balancing. A hand under the knees is very useful for this, or a hand on the middle of the back to help keep this straight.

8: Posture Sequences, Progression

Logical Posture Sequence

An experienced teacher can work out any number of graded sequences, keeping the general principles in mind.

The first posture in any sequence is usually simple forward flexing — this is a natural movement. The first postures are the standing ones; then lying; next the inverted. Back bends comes next, followed by twists and concluding with a repetition of the forward bends. Stronger movements come later in the sequence, when the muscles are thoroughly warmed and already well stretched. Early postures can be dynamic, to further the warming-up process.

The lying postures — second in the series — are both a preparation for inversion and a recuperation from the more tiring standing postures. Inversion (as in the Shoulder Stand) is followed by back bending, as with the Camel and the Cobra, to counter the stretching effect of this on the neck and shoulders. Any of the twists follow the backward bend and are themselves followed by the forward bending postures. (The back bends open the way for twists, as they involve the spinal muscles quite vigorously, while the twists loosen hips and shoulders — thus providing a preparation for the forward bends.) Twists must be followed by forward bends — the body requires straightening out!

It is not necessary to include all types of postures in one practice session or lesson — a sequence can be just lying, standing and sitting, using the lying postures as a preparation for the standing (see the sequence given in the section on the elderly, at the end of this chapter).

What must be remembered as an important principle is that for the physically handicapped who are not fit, there must be longer pauses than usual for relaxation between the postures. This is particularly true in the case of the elderly.

Choice of Postures

In Chapters Five, Six and Seven postures were roughly classified according to the action on the spine, i.e.

A   Straight spine
B   Flexed extended spine
C   Lateral flexion of spine
D   Twisting of spine
E   Inversion
F   More strenuous forms of any of these.

In each case some postures work minimally, others work extensively — obviously requiring more energy, more suppleness, and often greater physical ability to achieve the starting point. Also in each case postures are standing, sitting, kneeling or lying postures.

While sequences for handicapped people usually involve each category, the choice will be governed by the age, disability, disposition, and general physical fitness (or otherwise) of the pupil. The teacher needs to exercise care and skill in selecting the postures to use. With the physically handicapped — particularly spastic pupils — the fascinating thing is to see how more and more becomes possible. Postures become possible that were not even remotely imaginable in the early stages.

Sequences suitable for absolute beginners

It is easy to discourage people who are just starting yoga by what appears to them to be 'failure' — because they cannot achieve the finished posture as they see it, either as demonstrated or in pictures. It is therefore a good idea to give some extra time to the warming-up exercises, all or most of which are possible for practically everybody, whatever their age, physical condition or disability. In fact in some cases it may be as well to do *only* warming up exercises for the first few sessions, as these can bring about an improvement in the general physical condition. After this the teacher can introduce normal postures. This is particularly the case with the elderly.

Much of the practice or lesson time should be given over to breathing exercises, as the mastery of the breath is the greatest benefit of all to be gained from yoga.

Postures used should gently stretch the body—particularly the spine—in all directions, loosening areas where there is probably tension. At first the aim is to prepare the ground for getting into the correct starting position for subsequent, more complicated postures (see Chapters Five, Six and Seven):

Head Roll	No. A4	(Chapter Five)
Shoulder Roll	No. A6	(Chapter Five)
Eye Movements	No. A5	(Chapter Five)
Finger Stretch	No. A10	(Chapter Five)
Leg Loosener	No. A11	(Chapter Five)
Toe and Ankle Loosener	No. A12	(Chapter Five)
Half Moon	No. C2	(Chapter Seven)
Lion	No. A9	(Chapter Five)

Six of these eight postures can be carried out by anybody, whether sitting on the floor, in a wheelchair, or on an ordinary chair. There are no contra-indications. For a very handicapped person, a helper may be necessary to carry out the movement in the head and shoulder roll; a helper will most certainly be necessary for the Half Moon. Some version of the Pose of a Child (No. B20, Chapter Six), that is the Rag Doll version for those seated on chairs or in wheelchairs, or a forward crumpling version for those on the floor who cannot kneel, is possible to everybody. None of these postures involves much effort, but nor do they stretch the spine very effectively either.

The simplest of real spine-stretching exercises for people on the floor are:

Rabbit	No. B1	(Chapter Six)
Hare	No. B1	(Chapter Six)
Caterpillar	No. B3	(Chapter Six)
Spine flexion	No. B6	(Chapter Six)
Pose of Child	No. B19	(Chapter Six)
Cat	No. B5	(Chapter Six)
Dog	No. E1	(Chapter Seven)
Beam	No. B9	(Chapter Six)
Coil	No. B15	(Chapter Six)
Slow Roll	No. B16	(Chapter Six)

Except for the Beam and the Pose of a Child, these do not involve kneeling. They are not as difficult as those poses which involve sitting back on the heels — this requires flexible knee joints. Wheelchair or chair people can perform a version of the Cat, using a second chair in front of them, which is particularly useful for them as they almost never arch their backs. The Dog involves standing with the hands and feet on the floor, but it can be approached from a simple kneeling position, or from the Cat, so that people who cannot stand upright can still achieve it, particularly with help. The Beam involves kneeling with one leg out in front but a wall can be used as support. (Many spastic pupils can neither stand nor kneel.)

With the performance of all or some of these, the spine has been well flexed forward. For backward extension of the spine it is necessary to try:

Bridge	No. B10	(Chapter Six)
Camel	No. B11	(Chapter Six)
Cobra	No. F6	(Chapter Seven)

It is always possible to make some attempt at the Cobra, and the Bridge too — provided the knees bend; from the beginning a start may be made towards the Camel (for any who can kneel) simply by kneeling up and leaning back, without necessarily getting the hands as far as the ankles (a movement of which the pupil may be afraid). When first the ankle is reached (in the early stages), it is as well to grasp one ankle only and hold this, then return to the starting point; next leaning back to grasp the other — but not the two together. A pupil sitting on an ordinary chair, or better still a backless stool, can try this with the hand going to another chair behind. This again is excellent — people sitting in wheelchairs rarely flex their spines forward, and still more rarely extend them backwards.

For a twisting exercise to the spine, almost any of the poses — or some part of them as described in Chapter Seven — can be used. A good deal of the whole C section is within the reach of physically handicapped people.

The Simple Sitting Twist can be performed sitting on the floor, in a wheelchair, or on a chair: the legs should just be crossed over each other at the knee if possible, though this may well have to be done by the helper. If even this is not possible, a reasonable twist can still be obtained if the helper pushes or pulls the legs in the opposite direction from that of the arms and the trunk.

The Leg-over pose does twist the spine, particularly if the helper makes sure that the shoulders are flat on the ground. It is possible to hold the outstretched leg across in the air with one hand, and press down with the other hand just below the armpit on the opposite side, keeping the side of the chest well down.

For beginners who can stand, it is suitable to use:

Erect Posture	No. A1	(Chapter Five)
Tree	No. A10	(Chapter Five)
Side Stretch	No. C1	(Chapter Seven)
Back Stretch (Standing)	No. B8	(Chapter Six)

None of these is overtiring, as are many of the other standing poses, which prove to be suitable only for the fit.

Once confidence has been gained in these very simple poses, almost all of which are certainly possible to people on the floor, and many to people in wheelchairs, it is time to move on, as and when possible, to the more difficult ones, integrating them one at a time, and always introducing them in the middle of a session, when the muscles are thoroughly warmed and working to maximum capacity for the individual. The actual disability rules out some postures: for example, many spastics can neither stand nor kneel, nor can most people with spina bifida.

A Gentle Sequence

This would be suitable for the still-not-very-fit confined to the floor. If the pupils can stand, then the bracketed poses could be included. The change from the previous very simple posture sequences given would be very gradual — and it would depend entirely upon the individual which of the new postures were introduced first and which last. This following sequence could also be carried out by elderly people, always provided that any definite contra-indications were observed. The postures in brackets can be omitted to shorten the sequence.

Collecting into oneself
Warming up exercises
Leg Loosener   A11
(Erect Posture)   A1
(Tree)   A16
Cat   B5
Dog   E1
Cobra   F6
Swan   B4
Child   B19
Head Roll   A4
Head of Cow   A8
Cobbler   B18
(Triangle)   F3
Sitting Twist   D2
Plough or Half Shoulder Stand   E4
Pose of Child again
Alternate nostril breathing
Relaxation/meditation

A Sequence for the Fit
This series should satisfy even a highly active mentally handicapped youngster, if taken not too slowly with plenty of
energy given to warming up. It is not suitable for the
elderly — except the really experienced.

Collecting into oneself
Warming up exercises
Erect Posture   A1
Triangle   C4
Back Stretch, standing   B8
Spinal Flexion   B6 standing, and carried further than in
the description in Chapter 6.
Dancer   F1
Camel   B11
Pose of a Child   B19
Archer   B7
Sitting Twist   D2
Head of Cow   A8
Cobra   F6
Swan   B4

Cat   B5
Plough   E4
Back Stretch, sitting — dynamic version   B8
Fish   B12
Head Roll   A4
Floor   A18
Breathing, relaxation/meditation

A rather similar useful sequence would be:

Collecting into oneself
Alternate nostril breathing
Warming up, including the 'Ha' breath
Tree   A16
Triangle   F3
Reverse Triangle   F4
Back Stretch, sitting   B8
Cobra   F6
(Locust)   F9
(Bow)   F7
Plough   E4
Spinal Twist   D2
Head Roll   A4
Shoulder stand   E3
Bridge or Fish   B10, B12
Relaxation, breathing/meditation

What follows is a simple but rather less strenuous sequence, suitable for those who can stand.

Collecting of self
Warming up, including 'Ha' breath
Erect Posture   A1
Standing Back Stretch   B8
Triangle   F3
Squat   F5
Straight Leg over   D7
Coil   B15
Shoulder Stand and Plough   E3, E4
Cobra — counterpose to Plough   F6
Pose of Child — as counterpose to Cobra   B19
Sitting Twist   D2
Sitting Back Stretch   B8

Bridge   B10
Floor   A10
Breathing
Relaxation/Meditation

*Modifications for those with Downs Syndrome or those who
are mentally handicapped to any degree*
Here the important thing is to make the yoga fun (at this
point in the chapter, double disabilities, that is those with a
mental handicap who are also physically handicapped, are
excluded, as in this case the physical disability determines the
shape of the lesson).

It is as well to do very little breathing work at the
beginning: just a short while on the breathing of relaxation,
the breathing of action, reverting to the breathing of relaxation again, and then go through the warming up exercises
fully, but fairly fast. Demonstration is better than wordy
explanation, as the latter may not be listened to, while the
movements will be watched and can be imitated. Since these
people are not physically handicapped, the session can start
with some standing postures. Head and Shoulder Roll, Eye
movements could be found dull, not exciting enough, but
these four are quite strenuous enough:

The Tree	No. A10	(Chapter Five)
Triangle	No. C3	(Chapter Six)
Side Stretch	No. C2	(Chapter Seven)
Reverse Triangle	No. C4	(Chapter Six)

The difficulties of balancing in the Tree will cause fun. As
far as the Triangle and the Reverse Triangle are concerned,
it is better not to linger too long on the finer points. When
sitting down, the Back Stretch should be tried after easier
poses like the Cat, and countered by the Camel and the
Bridge. The Woodlouse is usually very much enjoyed and can
lead to the Cobra and Locust, while the Bow, more taxing
than either of these, is again exciting. The Plough should be
introduced before the half or whole Shoulder Stand, but all
three can be undertaken. Inverted poses give great pleasure
and a feeling of triumph and achievement, as does the Spinal
Twist.

None of the poses described are actually contra-indicated,

but the idea must be to provide pleasure, excitement and a sense of achievement. A youngster with Downs Syndrome will sometimes amaze and provoke envy in a teacher by proceeding into a full Lotus position without any apparent difficulty — even a bound Lotus!

With mentally handicapped people it is important that the warming-up process should be sufficiently vigorous to use a little of their latent energy, otherwise the whole practice session may prove somewhat restless and jerky. If they have been sufficiently stretched and made to achieve throughout, they will be quite happy to relax and follow a simple imaginative meditation at the end.

As previously stated, where there is double disability — both physical and mental — then the physical condition is bound to be the deciding factor in the poses and the general organisation of the session. Even so, the fun, interest and achievement factors must be borne in mind continually.

Progression
There is no special point in aiming for complex postures — indeed, none of the more complicated ones have been described. The whole value lies in gentle stretching and holding: this is how all the internal organs are stimulated and their functioning improved. Where there is disability, progress often comes not through mastering a pose perfectly, but through seeing a method of tackling a hitherto untried pose, with some modification perhaps of the starting point or with some additional help. It is possible to list the poses in each category as either simple or somewhat more strenuous:

Simple	*More Strenuous*
A	A
Simple Erect	Reclining Hero
Head Movements	Roll Twist
Head Roll	
Shoulder Roll	
Eye Movements	B
Cow's Head	Tree
Lion	Archer
Leg Loosener	Back Stretch

Simple	*More Strenuous*
A	**B**
Toe and Ankle Loosener	Beam
Hero	Camel
	Fish
	Moon
B	Platform
	Archer
Rabbit	Woodlouse
Hare	
Caterpillar	
Swan	
Cat	
Spinal Flexion	**C**
Bridge	
Chest Stretch	Rishi
Coil	Triangle
Slow Roll	Reverse Triangle
Cobbler	
Pose of Child	
Rag Doll	
	D
	Straight legs to floor
C	Leg Over
Side Stretch	Dynamic Twist
Half Moon	
D	**E**
Simple Standing Twist	Shoulder Stand
Spinal Stretch	
Lying Twist series	
Knee Chest Twist	
E	**F**
Dog	Cobra
Half Shoulder Stand	Locust
Plough	Bow

Progress is not measured by doing the more difficult pose though, nor in reaching further down or bending further back. It lies in the overall effect of yoga on the individual, that is the improvement not only in their fitness but also in the quality of their daily life, awareness, appreciation, response to emotional or environmental stress. As yoga becomes a way of life a tranquillity develops, a deep-rooted serenity and an ability to withstand stress. Above all the pupil acquires an ability to *enjoy*. Physical benefits are seen in much improved breath control, hence more energy, vitality, freedom from colds, extra suppleness and flexibility, particularly of the spine, and a generally improved circulation.

Where yoga is started reasonably young and kept up, the spine will not stiffen and arthritis will not come. This can be of immeasurable value to spastics and others with congenital disabilities. Due to the disability and resulting restricted and awkward movements, spinal and joint problems tend to come upon them early in life, leading to an early and unnecessary deterioration in their physical condition and so to a shorter life span than need be.

Chair work
As far as possible everybody should work from the floor. Many people however need to work from a chair at first, until they have built up their confidence. People who spend most of their days in wheelchairs feel singlularly vulnerable out of the chair to start with, and this advance should not be forced upon them before they are ready for it. Those with muscular dystrophy, except in the early stages, always get better breathing control if they are in their chairs where the chest is freer to expand, though a certain time should be spent on the floor to straighten the spine.

Work in a chair can include the warming-up exercises, also all the poses concerned with the top half of the body, such as the Head Roll, Shoulder Roll, Eye Movements, Lion, Head of Cow. The Half Moon can be done with the body and one arm tipping over the side of the chair. The Spinal Twist can be done crossing the legs if possible, otherwise with help to push the legs away from the side to which the body is turned. The Rag Doll version of the Pose of the Child simply involves collapsing forward like a rag doll with very little stuffing in it — arms hanging loosely down to the floor. If the legs can be raised in the wheelchair to rest on another chair in front, then a version of the Back Stretch (sitting) can be performed. A person sitting on a stool can do backwards stretching to a chair just behind, as a modification of the Fish. The rule of bending and stretching the spine in all directions in turn should be followed, however simply — even though the person is confined to a wheelchair.

Sequences confined to Floor

All postures except standing ones can be attempted on the floor, so the three basic rules to be followed are:

a) Exercise the spine in all directions, i.e. forward, back, sideways, twisting;

b) Follow pose by counterpose;

c) Keep milder movements to the beginning part of the lesson and do any more strenuous ones when every muscle has already been warmed in the early part.

Warming-up must involve work with arms, then legs, then whole body; breathing must have the relaxed breath and the action breath included; then simple postures are introduced such as Rabbit, Hare, Cat — the first two bending the spine forward, the Cat bending it both forward and backward, to be followed by the Bridge, which arches it well backwards, and perhaps the Leg Over as an easy twist.

The Sitting Back Stretch, combined with the Fish, the Bow and the Dynamic Twist form a more strenuous series still.

The Role of Helpers

One to a few

The helper needs to do just enough and not more — moving the paralysed arm in unison with the good one; lifting the elbows; straightening a contracted elbow joint; raising shoulders for breathing; helping back flexion by easing the trunk forward at the hips; rolling the head to make the movement generally bigger in the Head Roll; crossing one leg over the other in the Twist; extending the back in the Cobra by raising the upper half of the body; joining hands to heels in the Camel or Bow; and helping to lift the bottom off the floor in the Shoulder Stand or Plough; helping a person into the starting point for a posture, e.g. on to the knees; supporting the crossed leg in the

Leg Over, and keeping it crossed over at as high a level as possible. Provided the postures are taken slowly and held, one helper can often manage two or even three people in a session.

One to one
This is necessary when the pupil has any real degree of athetoid movements. The helper has to anchor the feet in any movement from lying to sitting, or sitting back down to lying; has to pause, hold the arms steady every few inches when movement is involved, until the spasm subsides; she will always need to keep the outstretched leg straight in the Leg Over (by standing with one foot against it while using both hands to support the other leg). In the Plough and Shoulder Stand, she needs to use her body as a support, having 'taken the pupil up', and she needs to be particularly careful to see that the 'coming down' is very gentle and smooth, with the back unfolding piece by piece—this actually requires both skill and strength.

Two to one
When a pupil is more or less totally paralysed—either through brain or spinal cord damage—or has the lack of control which results either from extreme spasticity or uncontrolled athetoid movements, it is necessary to have a helper on either side, so that every movement can be done for the pupil. The limits are 1) the degree of spasticity, which may be difficult to overcome; 2) the degree of joint immobility, which may have resulted over the years—which can *not* be overcome because of pain; 3) the weight of the person; and 4) the strength and stamina of the helper! The value to the pupil is literally enormous, even though he has to be entirely passively moved. He gets a stimulation, massaging, squeezing and relaxing of the abdominal organs that he never gets in the normal way.

The Elderly
Problems that may be present in elderly people—apart from some definite disability—are stiffness, lack of flexibility, lack of strength, diminished breathing capacity, worsening circulation, varicose veins, poor balance, fatigue due to lessened

breathing capacity and impaired circulation, weakened digestion, tendency to bowel trouble, memory impairment,
inability to concentrate, lower back weakness and foot trouble
(flat feet, bunions, corns.)

Disabilities are likely to be:

Residual paralysis of some degree following a stroke;
Osteoarthritis of hips and knees;
Some degree of spinal arthritis, particularly in the neck;
Chronic sinusitis, bronchitis;
Congestive heart failure;
High blood pressure;
Low blood pressure.

One of the first difficulties that arises is the attitude of mind of
the elderly person. This is likely to be compound of self
consciousness, trepidation in case the lesson is too difficult or
too exhausting, and doubt as to whether there is 'anything in
yoga anyway'.

If the prospective pupil is very timorous, it may be a good
idea to let him sit on a chair and watch for the first session,
joining in a breathing exercise or two, trying the Half Moon,
Head and Shoulder Rolls and Rag Doll. Probably other
equally elderly pupils can reassure him more than the teacher.
Self-consciousness passes off after a time or two, as none of the
older hands are self-conscious. The doubt disappears even
more rapidly when the improvement in general well-being
becomes evident, which it does very quickly.

Actually a person is never too stiff or too old to begin the
practice of yoga, and yoga slows the aging process by its beneficial effect on breathing, circulation and the suppleness of the
spine. 'You are as young as your spine is flexible.' Because
everyone has problems, the elderly may fit in quite well in any
class for handicapped people, where the pace is slower and the
work generally less strenuous than in an ordinary class. The
ordinary one-and-three-quarter-hour class with normal
younger people can prove so exhausting for the older person
that he is put off at once and never returns. This takes place
no matter how much the teacher may advise the student not to
do too much, not to get overtired, to stop as soon as he has had
enough etc. He does not know *in time* that he has had enough,
or that he is overtired, and consequently he is left at the end of

the class with a flat feeling of exhaustion instead of a sense of well-being—and can even feel worse the next day. Better ten times too slow and easy at the start than one single degree too fast.

The initial aims should be to teach breath control (improving what are probably the faulty breathing practices of a lifetime), to bring some added flexibility to the spine, and to teach relaxation. (It is taken for granted that the teacher has found out what specific problems, if any, her elderly pupils have and, roughly at least, their ages. Seventy to seventy-five seems to be the watershed—below this the pupil is 'Young Elderly' and above it, 'Elderly, Elderly'. But it is possible for some people in their sixties to be already 'Elderly Elderly', both in body and in mind! 'Elderly Elderlies' have to be dealt with much more carefully—remembering that their stamina is much lower than that of the 'Young Elderly'.

A class of about forty minutes is enough to start with: ten minutes on breathing in the Relaxation pose, with some arm and leg movements, moving on to the Bridge pose; three minutes on some of the warming up exercises, carried out lying down (excluding rolling probably), then fifteen minutes on Rabbit, Hare, Cat—that is forward flexion of the spine—, Camel (modified version)—that is extension of the spine—, Simple Twist or one of the twists lying, and slow Spinal Roll—which is almost the movement that comes at the beginning of an inverted posture such as the Plough. Finally five to ten minutes' relaxation—with a simple concentration exercise like the Canoe or Cloud (see Chapter Ten).

After this very easy programme no one will feel exhausted or overwhelmed, and the teacher will have been able to see how great the breathing problems are, and the degree of stiffness of the spine. Other poses that may be introduced over the next few sessions would be the Erect or Standing pose, Head Roll, Shoulder Roll, Eye Movements, Tree, Lion and Standing Half Moon, Head of Cow in Thunderbolt or Hero Position, Backstretch standing and sitting, also the other lying Spinal Twists.

Stronger standing poses like the Triangle and Reverse Triangle are better left until the pupils are themselves stronger—the older age group may never reach postures of this strength—; the Cobra comes earlier than the Locust and the Bow; the Plough comes before the Shoulder Stand: but both must be embarked upon rather cautiously. A good preparation for the inverted poses in the elderly is to get them to lie on their backs, with the bottom close to a wall, then lift their legs up the wall. This is good for the blood flow in the legs, moreover the legs can be brought off the wall over towards the head, knees and ankles together, and then the knees flexed on to the chest. After some weeks of doing this, the pupil's hands, or a helper's hands, can help the bottom a little way up off the floor—and the result is a considerable way towards the Half Shoulder Stand, brought about very easily and devoid of trauma or anxiety.

With the use of the stronger sitting and lying poses, the abdominal viscera are greatly toned, digestive difficulties are lessened, liver and pancreatic function improved, bowel functioning stimulated; all this contributes greatly to the overall improvement in health, renewed zest for living and generally 'younger look'.

Until a degree of strength is acquired, no pose should be held for a long time, and the standing poses should be used very sparingly. It is very difficult for a fit young yoga teacher to envisage quite how tiring standing postures are for elderly people. Careful monitoring of the breathing of her pupils should however make her aware of it—audible gasps, ragged breathing, grunts at the end of expiration, are sure signs that the elderly pupil is being overtaxed. The 'just' elderly, without any additional disability, are unlikely to require helpers, though some of the aids cited could be very useful in the early stages.

Where there is additional disability, this has to be the prime consideration in the choice of posture, and may well necessitate the pupil spending his session in a chair, at any rate to start with.

None of the postures in this book are unsuitable for the elderly, unless they have one or other of the specific disabilities. The general improvement in breathing and circulation is remarkable, and, together with the regained flexibility of the spine, brings about a great improvement in general health. Also the ability to concentrate on the postures increases steadily, and this spills over into daily life so that memory improves, and vagueness, even disorientation, can improve too.

A simple session for the unfit.
Collecting into self.
Breathing and relaxation.
Action breath.
Addition of arms to action breaths.
Coil **B15**
Simple spinal Roll **B16** Chapter Six
Balancing with simple movements of one leg, Chapter Three.
Warming up **A6 A7 A8**
Erect Posture, drop forward by weight.
Swinging with hips in dropped over position.
Unrolling to the erect position vertebra by vertebra, head last.
Dropping again, and unrolling bringing the head first.
Opening and closing movements, first the hands, then arms opening out, slightly sideways, then involving the shoulders, finally the head — up and back — to full posture of receptivity.
Spinal Twist, lying, Chapter Seven **D4** The following four versions:
a. Foot on top of other foot.
b. Foot on knee.
c. Feet side by side apart, close to the buttocks.
d. Feet side by side, together, close to the buttocks.
Lie with bottom close to wall, lift feet on to the wall spread legs wide.
Lie on side, with the underneath knee slightly bent, bring the second foot over on top of the knee and put the underneath hand on this knee. Carry out sweeping circles, backwards, upwards, then down in front of the face with the uppermost arm, following the arm with head and eyes.
Change, and repeat on the other side.
Repeat the Coil.
Breathing of relaxation.
Some simple meditation from among the first five to be found in Chapter Ten.

Taken slowly, this sequence is possible even for the unfit elderly. After a few weeks, the pupil should have improved sufficiently to tackle the next sequence.

Another simple sequence
This will not take very long and will not overstrain. It is suit-

able for the elderly unless they are very unfit, also for those physically handicapped who can stand. It is not strenuous or exciting enough for fit mentally handicapped youngsters.

> Collection of self.
> Breathing of relaxation.
> Breathing of Action.
> Simple Spinal Stretch.
> Coil.
> Bridge.
> Cat.
> Dog.
> Half Moon: Standing.
> Rishi's posture.
> Sitting back stretch.
> Cobra.
> Floor posture.
> Relaxation meditation, from Chapter Ten.

And a Third

Here is another sequence suitable for elderly people, when they have acquired a little experience and are generally fitter — it will be noted that the nearest to an inverted pose is the Dog.

> Collection of self
> Breathing of relaxation and of action
> Warming up
> Coil **B15**
> Straight leg over **D7**
> Knees to chest Spinal Twist **D5**
> Dog **E1**
> Tree **A16**
> Standing Back Stretch **B8**
> Pose of Child **B19**
> Bridge
> Spinal Roll

If standing is too strenuous, then the Cat, **B5** the Swan, **B4** and the sitting Back Stretch could be substituted for the Tree and the standing Back Stretch.

With regard to the elderly who have definite disabilities, advice to help with their problems is to be found in Chapter Nine.

9: Specific Disabilities

One of the most important principles to be observed in dealing with handicapped people is—not to concentrate on the handicap. Yoga is for the whole person, body, mind and spirit and the tendency to treat a stiff back, arthritis, scoliosis etc. must be avoided. If there is a disability, certain postures may be specially helpful, and others are distinctly contra-indicated, but the whole body must be stretched, toned, made more flexible. Slow working, plenty of relaxation and moderation are the key notes—and every degree of physical disability, including old age, will benefit. (As already pointed out in Chapter Eight, sessions with the mentally handicapped are different).

An intuitive teacher can find innumerable small variations that add to the value, demands and interest of the very simplest of postures, when she is dealing with somebody who is either very frail or very incapacitated.

Asthmatics and Those with Other Chest Conditions

Many of these may be confined to chairs. Others, when they are put on to the floor cannot lie on their face nor flat on their back, but have to be well propped up on cushions. This limits the poses that are possible. On the other hand, people with chest conditions benefit tremendously if considerable attention is paid to the breathing side of the programme. But even here advances must be slow, most particularly in the realm of retention after inhalation— this must not be attempted for a considerable time.

Plenty of time must be given to the relaxed breath with only the abdomen moving; stress should be laid on the accompanying relaxation of face and shoulders—the latter helping greatly in asthmatic problems—and the absence of the need for any positive effort on inspiration, just letting the air come in when it wants to, effortlessly. Mastery of the relaxed breath is the key to success with asthmatic sufferers. Only after this has been mastered—and it will probably take several sessions—should the action breath be considered, and then those movements that go to open up the lungs—arm-raising etc.

Postures of special value for those with breathing difficulties—particularly asthmatics—are the Bridge, the Hero, Half Moon, Reclining Hero, the Platform and the Fish. All of these work by stretching the chest muscles in the actual posture, so that the movements of respiration stretch them still more (needless to say they *must not* be attempted if the chest is at all in spasm). The Rabbit, Hare, Caterpillar and Spinal Stretch are also very useful in these *and* other chest conditions, and should be practised before poses where the chest is compressed are tackled, because in each of them a different lobe of the lung is free to work, the movement of the others being restricted. Further to these, other poses such as the Head of Cow, Cobra, Locust and Bow can all be introduced. However, the ability to perform these last does depend, to some extent, on the underlying cause of the chest trouble. Eventually these people can work against chest compression as in the Dog, Shoulder Stand and Plough, Dynamic Back Stretch and Sitting Twist. The Dynamic Back Stretch should be attempted in the version with the foot in the groin and the hand outstretched to the opposite foot.

Cardiac Conditions—such as congenital heart lesions, valvular disease of the heart, congestive heart failure etc.
Some—perhaps most—of these students also come into the previous category, since they also have breathing difficulties and are unable to lie flat on the floor. If they can lie down, care must be taken to avoid making them breathless. That means that all postures must be taken at a very slow pace, and none should be used where inhalation has to work against any degree of restriction,—as in the Twists—particularly the Sitting Twists. Many people with heart conditions do a considerable amount of abdominal breathing, keeping their chests rigid and immovable. In this case, the preliminary exercises are very important, particularly the breathing of relaxation. It may take several sessions to overcome the tension present in the chest and shoulders, and to master the breath-

ing of relaxation before moving on to the breath of action.

The series of arm movements added to the action breath are very useful taken next, while simple subsequent postures are Rabbit, Hare, Caterpillar, Spinal Stretch, Beam, Cat and Dog, then Hero and the other chest stretching ones like the Bridge. The Camel and Fish may always prove too strenuous. The Cobra is a possibility, and of course all the earlier simple postures, such as the Shoulder Roll, Head Roll, Eye Movements, Finger Stretch, Lion etc.

A simple safe rule to follow where there is congenital heart disease or valvular disease is that the pupil must not be allowed to become breathless; he must perform within the limitations of his breathing ability. A person with congestive heart failure — already breathless — should work only on the breathing, and do no poses.

Where there is a history of coronary thrombosis (myocardial infarction), the thing to bear in mind is that once the initial period of intensive care is over and the subsequent few weeks of gradually increasing exercise have taken place, then a scar has been formed in the damaged heart muscle. Subsequent exercising to improve the coronary circulation and strengthen the heart muscle is wholly good, and the pupil will benefit enormously from steadily developing exercises. In the same way a person with angina can benefit from yoga — always keeping well short of the postures that might produce cardiac pain. There are plenty of non-strenuous yoga postures. Many of the ones described in this book are no more taxing than walking about — but are of much more value to the circulation!

People with palpitations, that is occasional outbursts of undue and uncomfortable consciousness of the heart beating, can take any fairly easy sequence and also seem to be helped by the standing Back Stretch and the Reclining Hero, though these should not be included if there is also high blood pressure.

Strokes

People who have had strokes will also benefit greatly from yoga, even though they may require a lot of help if they have a paralysed side. Of particular value are the simple poses: Head Roll and Shoulder Roll; and chest openers such as Half Moon, Head of Cow and Twist. Usually the kneeling postures are out;

the Cobra, with its flushing effect on the kidneys is of great value, while the Posterior Stretch and Bridge — if the latter can be managed — keep the spine flexible. For people whose blood pressure is high, the Plough, the Back Stretch, sitting, (including the dynamic version) and the Hero are all valuable; also, most particularly, the floor postures. The Half Shoulder Stand is fine, but the Full Shoulder Stand is better avoided. The Dog makes the simplest inverted posture. Otherwise none of the poses, provided it is possible to do, is contra-indicated. Often a pupil may show some resistance to any poses that look strenuous, due to fear, in which case it is as well not to over-persuade stroke patients to do them. Use encouragement, but no pressure. For instance, very often it takes quite a while for a stroke person to be persuaded out of a chair and on to the floor. There is no hurry — they can get tremendous benefit working in a wheelchair, then an ordinary chair, then possibly on a backless stool, or straight on to the floor — well propped up and well helped! It does not matter if it takes months before this stage is reached — nor if it never is.

Epileptics

There is no reason why people with epilepsy should not tackle any of the poses. Breathing and relaxation exercises are of great value, but care should be taken over retention after inhalation, and holding after exhalation. Perhaps one particular posture that ought to be avoided would be the Eye Movements exercise; if done vigorously this might, in some cases, trigger off a convulsion. In the early stages, postures compressing the chest should also be left out of the sequences, and care should always be taken not to have an over-vigorous session. The teacher will 'feel' her way somewhat, as will the student. People with epilepsy can often monitor their own condition, and if the student feels it is a bad day for him, or that a fit might be coming on, it would be as well to let him do nothing but simple breathing exercises and a great deal of relaxation. Any attempt to 'work it off' must be strongly discouraged — this does not happen. The Plough is to be preferred to the Shoulder Stand and the Quick Roll is perhaps better left out. On the other hand a well controlled epileptic, where some time has elapsed since he had an attack, should not in any way be singled out from the ordinary. Occasional 'petit mal' attacks during a session are no indication for stopping.

Spastics (Cerebral Palsy)

People who have cerebral palsy are likely to form a majority in any class for physically handicapped people. Their handling depends largely upon the degree of disability, and to a lesser degree upon their age. For those with very little disability, all the postures described are possible. For clarity, four different types of cerebral palsy are considered here, but obviously all variations and degrees will be met.

1) A walking spastic person of over middle age probably has a very stiff spine, fixed in a somewhat hyperextended posture. Standing postures here will not meet with much success, and all work should be carried out on the floor. The student should be encouraged to lie on his back. The tendency will be to turn on his side, in view of the arching back, so a great deal of time must be spent on simple back flexion postures: Rabbit, Hare, Caterpillar, Cat, Sitting Back Stretch. The Cobra may cause the back to 'lock', but the Locust is a possibility as a counterpose to forward flexion. If a reasonable sitting position is attainable on the floor, then the Archer is an excellent pose to attempt, however unsuccessfully, while the Coil, Plough and Shoulder Stand all help. Extreme care must be taken in coming out of the Shoulder Stand — the spine tends to move in one solid piece, putting a very great strain on the lumbosacral region. This strain can be largely avoided if the student is told to bend the head forward on coming out, contrary to the teaching for a class of fit people. The younger the spastic, the less likely is it for the spine to have become rigid. A much greater range of postures may be tackled with young pupils.

2) Spastics with a paralysed side, arm and leg, but perhaps with a back less rigid than the group described above (especially if they are young) can *attempt* all postures described except the standing ones, though some are likely to be very minimally achieved. In all probability there is no adequate shoulder movement on the paralysed side — limiting the Shoulder Roll, for instance —, and the arm on that side will need help to reach up over the head, as in the Sitting Half Moon or Sitting Back Stretch. The Head of a Cow will pose problems too, while the Sitting Twist proves much more diffi-

cult on one side, with no good arm and shoulder movement possible backwards. Very probably too in such a pupil the legs will not flex at the knee. This limits the Coil, Cobbler, Roll, Woodlouse, Shoulder Stand and Bow on the one hand, and (because of the inability to kneel) the Rabbit, Hare, Caterpillar and Cat on the other. These poses, other than the kneeling ones, the Coil etc. — can however be attempted with help. It is surprising how far such a youngster can get with a Shoulder Stand, also with help, and the Plough, and he will gain great personal satisfaction.

3) When dealing with a young spastic person with athetoid movements, but no paralysis, it is essential in all movements into and out of poses to pause at each step until the 'shakes' have steadied. A very small movement-under-control is worth waiting for. On the other hand, too much of this can make the session incredibly dull, and an 'all out' attack at more exciting postures, in spite of terrific jerking, has its part to play in keeping the student happy. Very often, spastics of this ilk are found to be more controlled in the inverted postures, and hence get great pleasure from them. All poses can be attempted, except probably the standing ones. Such a student may be able to do everything on the floor except kneel, which then rules out all the postures with that as a starting point (the ability to kneel may come after some considerable time, even after several years spent on other poses). One difficulty with athetoid spastic people seems to be that very often they have no idea how to use their arms as a support, and this takes a long time to teach. This particular group is one of the most rewarding to deal with, however, as the progress the student makes can be phenomenal — the advent of control, of improved position, of real spinal flexibility, is heart-warming. The teacher finds herself saying — 'If only I had got hold of him earlier'. This is equally true of the older spine-stiffened spastic person. His situation deteriorates so much as the spine becomes more rigid.

4) If coping with a spastic person who has no controlled movements, or practically none, every movement has to be done for him. Much depends on the severity of the spasticity, and the age at which he starts yoga, as to how much or how little can be accomplished. If put on the floor, such a spastic person can be put through a range of movements at every

joint. Thus does not seem much to resemble yoga, but during this exercise the pupil can *think* into every movement, and may even develop a slight element of control here and there (miracles cannot be expected). However, the improvement in the breathing pattern, at the end of a yoga session, if the teacher has carried out the movements and the pupil has done the thinking, is truly amazing. And to slow the breathing pattern in a severely spastic boy, who literally wears himself out with his rapid breathing rate hour after hour, is worth a great deal. (Much easier to help than this spastic form of para-lysis, is the flaccid paralysis of someone who has had polio.)

Due to their very spasticity, all spastic people tend to have chests full of tension, even those with quite a mild degree of spasticity. The degree of tension can often be noted by the rapidity of the respiratory rate, produced by the restricted movement of a rigidly held chest and resulting in deficient air intake and so oxygen shortage.

Spina Bifida

Many people with spina bifida are magnificent from the waist up; with head, trunk and arms they can do anything, and they can usually move their legs by hand into any position. Standing positions are not possible, unless thay are wearing callipers, although if helped into position they may achieve the Dog, with a slightly precarious balance. Some can achieve a kind of kneeling posture, which is worth building on, but this is only possible for forward movements, as in the Cat, not for sitting back. It has to be remembered that there is virtually no weight in the bottom part of the body: overbalancing is easy. Others may have arm weakness as well, and hydrocephalus is a common accompaniment; such a pupil may or may not have some form of valve in situ. In such a pupil, the spine tends to move 'en masse', and depending upon the type and actual site of the reparative operations of infancy, it is very difficult for him to unfold his spine on to the floor, vertebra by vertebra. Consequently this simple exercise in spine flexibility is well worth practising in order to achieve such flexibility as proves to be possible. Shoulder Stands are not possible—because of the leg paralysis the pupil goes automatically, and with no difficulty into the Plough. For poses like the Simple Twist, he can 'place' his legs carefully into position manually. In the

Cobra the lack of back flexibility shows very clearly; almost in-
evitably he will bring the hips off the ground, so the teacher
has to be content with very little uplift; any 'nip' in the back at
waist level is a minor triumph.

A person who has hydrocephalus accompanying his spina
bifida can do any pose within the limitations imposed by his
legs: the head makes no difference. Where there is a valve in
situ, this too makes no difference—even the Plough can be
performed with no harm taken. Clearly, such a pupil, if
complaining of a headache, would not do any yoga at all,
other than relaxation and the simplest of breathing exercises,
with no retention or holding, and should already be receiving
a medical check.

Muscular Dystrophy

The comparatively rapid progress of this disease means that
these pupils very quickly have no muscular power worth speaking of, and almost every movement has to be done for them.
Apart from the steady deterioration, they resemble people
who have had polio (infantile paralysis), presenting the same
type of flaccid paralysis. They achieve a point of balance
sitting in a chair and do their best yoga from this position,
although in the very early stages they can go on to the floor
and make an attempt at all postures. Remembering that chest
trouble is their great danger, breathing exercises are an absolute essential for them. Some mastery of breath control may
well save their lives later on.

Particularly important are those breathing exercises which
open up the bottom of the lungs: forward arm raising and the
Half Moon; and the Shoulder lift, shaking the shoulders down
from the ears in a series of jerks, which forcibly expels air from
the lung bases. The helper probably needs to carry out all the
positive movements.

One result of lack of muscular power is the inability to raise
the head if it has dropped forward (or backwards). For
example, when the helper is bringing a pupil up after he has
collapsed forward in a Rag Doll position she must support the
head at the back with one hand—otherwise it will drop helplessly backwards with a most unpleasant jar.

As with all neuromuscular disorders, it is particularly
important in the case of muscular dystrophy to avoid fatigue.

The yoga teacher needs to be particularly vigilant with these pupils—they can be very determined, work too hard, and exhaust themselves. They must be convinced that it is not the degree of physical effort that counts.

Most of their work needs a helper on a one-to-one basis.

Degenerative Diseases of the Central Nervous System
i.e. Multiple Sclerosis, Cerebellar ataxia—for example —Friedreich's—and Parkinson's Disease.

Whatever the severity of the disease, when the person presents at a yoga class some postures can be found that can be achieved, perhaps without help, perhaps with a great deal of help. Yoga may do a great deal to build up the pupil's confidence and bring about a very real improvement.

There is no contra-indication in these diseases to putting the pupil on the floor and no contra-indication to any pose that proves to be even vaguely possible. Plenty of time must be allowed for the pupil's own efforts, before help is given. Conversely, sometimes if a pupil is helped into the starting point for the pose, he can carry on from there. A long period of time should be spent on breathing at the beginning of a session, to establish relaxed breathing and break down any barriers to the energy flow. In later stages of the disease it may be necessary to have two helpers to one pupil. Fatigue must be avoided, as it is definitely harmful.

People with Freidreich's ataxia often present when quite young, as the disease may show almost from birth. They have some degree of spastic paralysis, rather like the cerebral palsy pupils but with rather more difficulty of coordination. Again, breathing is very important, though they rarely have the same tension as the spastics. No poses are contra-indicated, they do whatever lies within their power. Later on, balance becomes a problem and all the work has to be carried out on the floor.

Yoga offers a great deal to people with multiple sclerosis. Again, the earlier they start the better. So much in MS depends upon the mental attitude of the person who has it. A chip on the shoulder, resentment, seems to inhibit recovery from the initial attack, which acquiescence, acceptance, with no determination to do one's best seems equally harmful. It is a disability in which there is often tremendous tension, blockage to the energy flow, inability to breathe properly—either the breathing of relaxation or of action. Many sessions can be spent on breathing alone, before any postures are attempted, and then these can be introduced gradually according to the physical state of the pupil. Since this is a deteriorating disease the pupil may have any degree of disability, from a little difficulty in walking and moderate arm weakness, to total paralysis of all four limbs, with respiratory muscles involved, and the muscles of swallowing. It does appear that regular yoga therapy can accelerate the improvements—it is a disease of exacerbations and remissions—and perhaps hold off the exacerbations. At any rate evidence is being accumulated that points in that direction. (It must be remembered that yoga is not just a form of physiotherapy—it is a way of life.)

People with Parkinson's disease usually present in older age groups than those with dystrophy or Friedreich's ataxia, or the more middle-of-life MS person. Consequently they present the usual problems of aging as well as those of the disease. The paralysis is a spastic one and they must work quietly within their capacity. It is very important to avoid fatigue and agitation—both make the condition much worse. The teacher has to bear in mind that the disease makes for slow reactions, but the intelligence is unimpaired, although the pupil may take a time to initiate a movement in response to any suggestion. This is characteristic—and one of the more depressing factors of the disease for the person who has it.

Motor Neurone Disease
Among degenerative diseases of the central nervous system, this needs special mention People with this disease may possibly present at a class, snatching at anything that might conceivably offer help. They should be allowed to try anything that seems possible—but must never make themselves breathless. Much time should be given to the breathing of relaxation, to overcoming tension, to relaxation proper and simple meditation. Their problem lies in the ultimate failure of the respiratory muscles.

Infantile Paralysis (poliomyelitis)
People who have had an attack of infantile paralysis are fortunate indeed, and rare, if they escape with absolutely no

impairment of their breathing, so one of the most valuable aspects of yoga for them is work on breath control. No postures are contra-indicated, it is just a question of the degree and sites of the muscular paralysis. The paralysis is flaccid and not spastic, so there is no resistance to the limbs being helped into any pose, and circulation is usually uniformly very poor, due to the lack of the stimulation that comes from natural muscular movement. All the organs benefit from the stimulation that follows when the pupil is literally lifted and put into the appropriate posture. Where breathing is very impaired, the pupil may be rather timid about going on to the floor, and may need to start in a chair, he will progress thence to the floor as confidence increases. Very often these pupils achieve the Lotus posture with no difficulty, and can do all their sitting work in this pose.

Absence of thigh muscles may make kneeling up difficult, and some postures may be completely impossible if the arms cannot be used as supports.

Rheumatoid Arthritis
People with Rheumatoid Arthritis should do nothing other than breathing exercises and relaxation during any acute flare-up. It must be remembered that Rheumatoid Arthritis is a general illness—it is not just applicable to the joints—and illness requires rest. Outside these times, all postures that are possible should be done—without strain (as always in yoga). Movement should stop short of pain in the affected joints—which are most likely to be the smaller joints, fingers, wrists, and elbows. If the knees are involved it is better to avoid the standing postures and to do everything that is possible lying down or sitting on the floor. When the joints have no weight-bearing to do, a rather greater range of movement is possible. Advanced cases will be confined to a wheelchair and require the maximum help for minimum movement, which must always be inside the edge of pain. People with Rheumatoid Arthritis almost always exhibit great tension, and steady work at relaxation is of the greatest help, with a great deal of attention to the breathing of relaxation.

Osteo-arthritis
These pupils are usually in older age groups. In the early

stages they benefit by all exercises. Frequently the overall improvement in circulation that results from yoga can produce a very dramatic improvement in the arthritic condition. This can remain permanent if yoga practice is persevered with. If starting at a later stage, then there are some changes which cannot be reversed—here the arthritic has to do his practising within the limits set by pain, but with steady regular practice the advance of the disease can be held in check. It is of great advantage to work regularly on the spine, so that this is kept flexible, even if knees and hips are stiff. No poses that can be attempted are contra-indicated.

Spinal Trouble

Yoga is not contra-indicated where there is trouble in the spine—quite the reverse. It is however very necessary to know what the lesion is, if any, where it is, and how chronic it is. Short of this knowledge it is as well to concentrate on breathing and relaxation—those simple arm movements which go to open up the lungs in breathing, and the minor spinal flexion exercises which cannot possibly do any harm, such as Head Roll, Shoulder Roll, Half Moon, Rabbit, Hare, Caterpillar, Cat, Dog, Bridge, Pose of Child, Spinal Flexion. If the lesion is known to be in the cervical area, the head should not be allowed to drop back in the Head Roll, and the squeeze back of the head in the second part of the Cat must also be avoided, ditto in the Cobra, though the rest of the spinal movement in this is excellent, as are also the Bridge, Bow, Fish and the first part of the Chest stretch.

The dorsal area is not usually affected, unless there is rigidity of the whole spine as in Ankylosing Spondylitis, of which more later. Most back troubles are in the lower back, and vary from muscular strain to prolapsed inter-vertebral disc or spinal arthritis. It is very important to know whether the disc has actually prolapsed or not, also if this is of long or short standing. Stiffness and muscular strain respond to slow gentle stretching of quite long duration, daily or twice daily, or even more frequently. It is as well to use simple poses that the pupil can carry on with on his own. There is no limit to the amount of time that can be spent on the exercises.

There is a variation of the locust specially good for low back pain, where the legs are bent at the knee, thighs kept apart, and shins perpendicular to the floor. On exhalation the thighs are lifted and brought together, while the shins remain perpendicular.

Where there is some disorganisation of the inter-vertebral joint, so that a disc lesion is threatened, the first thing that happens is that all the spinal muscles go into a protective spasm. This is what causes the pain. And this pain is best overcome by gentle stretching, utilising all those postures which stretch the muscles in the lower back area. It is essential that the body should be really warm before these are done, so in spite of stiffness and wariness about moving, the warming-up process is very very important. There should only be minimal movement in the opposite direction — that is, extension of the spine — but the Spinal Twist is quite safe to do. The exercises must be practised slowly, held for quite a time and repeated morning and evening, more if at all possible.

Where there has been a recent *proven* disc prolapse, stretching exercises are best; breathing with arms extended over head and legs stretched equally; the Bridge, with the feet well away from the buttocks so that the stretch on the spine is greater then the hyperextension; the Back Stretch, sitting, with the back stretched slowly and cautiously — particularly that version in which the head is kept up and the pupil holds on to the toes with arched back; and the first stage of the Cobra, a variation with the arms outstretched above the head, and raising from the floor *with* the head.

With chronic disc lesions the guiding note is pain. The pupil should exercise gently in all directions, stopping just short of pain, and holding each position for a longer period than usual. Wherever possible the force of gravity should be used to pull on the spine. All movements should be very slow and smooth — the pupil should be told to go to just the edge of pain and hold, coming out with equal slowness. It should be possible gradually to get further with each pose. Chronic disc lesions with pain of many years standing can greatly improve their range of movement with persistent practice of this type — always stopping short of real pain.

Ankylosing Spondylitis

In this disease the whole spine is affected. Here the guiding word is caution. Many of these people are on cortisone, which results, long term, in increasing the fragility of the bones. Breathing, relaxation and arm and leg movements are probably all that can be attempted, as the spine is likely not only to be rigid the whole way down but also extremely fragile.

Spinal arthritis
These people benefit greatly from regular yoga practice — using the simple poses to ensure flexibility before venturing on the more complex ones. The simple ones have the advantage of working only on one little bit of the spine at a time, and being easy. The more complex ones have the advantage of having a much stronger effect on all the internal organs as well as on the whole spine.

Low Blood Pressure
Whatever the cause of the low blood pressure, if the pupil is known to have it, he should do all his work on the floor, and be particularly careful when changing from lying to sitting, sitting to kneeling, kneeling back to kneeling up. The reason for this is that blood pressure falls each time with the position changing movements. This care should be observed with the elderly, whatever their blood pressure. Any posture producing breathlessness or rapid heartbeat should be avoided. Slow gentle work, with plenty of stretching, plenty of time between postures, and much time spent on breathing exercises is to be recommended.

Eye and Ear Troubles
Avoid inverted postures and the Woodlouse, otherwise everything is possible. If any posture produces a feeling of congestion in the head (the Triangle may), it is as well to leave it. The Back Stretch should only be performed sitting.

Palming — i.e. rubbing the hands together and then cupping them over the eyes, repeated several times — is of value, as is the Head Roll, Shoulder Roll and Head of Cow.

Gastric or Duodenal Ulcer
In sessions for a person suffering from an ulcer, most attention should be given to relaxation and breath control. A trigger factor with ulcers is the individual's high degree of tension. If this can be overcome, then the pupil is a long way towards

curing himself. All work should be carried out particularly slowly and calmly, the postures should be held for as long as possible, and great attention should be paid to the correct breathing throughout the whole posture: that is preparing for it, going into it, staying in it, and coming out of it. The pupil must always relax into the posture, and should not hold his breath. Dynamic postures should be avoided. When the ulcer is known to be active, inverted postures should be avoided, as should all postures compressing the gut. If the teacher feels it necessary to do at least one of these to maintain a balanced sequence, then it should be held only for a short time.

Diaphragmatic Hernia

If this is severe, all work must be carried out sitting in a chair and forward bending kept to a minimum. Even the collapse forward of the Rag Doll is too severe. Backward bending is possible. If work is carried out on the floor, the Cat and the Swan, all twists and backward bends are fine. If lying down postures are tried it is as well to prop the upper part of the body up on several cushions, reducing these as the condition appears to improve. In standing work all inverted postures must be avoided, and forward bending again kept to a minimum. Much time and attention should be given to breathing work to strengthen the diaphragm. In the early stages anything compressing the gut is best avoided.

Before working out sequences for people with the disabilities described in this chapter, reference should be made back to Chapters Five, Six, and Seven, where the postures carry details of their therapeutic value.

There follows a brief resumé of postures that have specific value in given disabilities.

Pupils with Asthma, Bronchitis, Lung Troubles
Initially Bridge, Half Moon, Hero and Reclining Hero. Then Rabbit, Hare, Caterpillar, Spinal Stretch, leading on to Camel, Fish and Platform. Next, Head of Cow, Cobra, Locust and Bow and finally Dog, Half Shoulder Stand and Plough, even the Sitting Twist.

Pupils with Cardiac Conditions
Rabbit, Hare, Caterpillar, as well as the Head Roll, Shoulder Roll, Finger Stretch. Then Spinal Stretch, Beam and Cat, leading on to the Dog, Hero and Reclining Hero, Bridge.

Stroke Pupils
Head Roll, Shoulder Roll, Finger Stretch, Half Moon, Head of Cow and Twists. Then Cobra, Posterior Stretch, and Bridge. Even the half shoulder stand, *if* preceded by the Plough.

Osteoarthritis of Hips and knees
Cobbler, Hero—gradually; Archer—very gradually; ordinary cross legged sitting.

Osteoarthritis of Shoulder
Particularly the Shoulder Roll, Head of Cow, Front Stretch, and Spinal Stretch.

Cervical Disc
Head movement—not backwards—, Shoulder Roll, Half Moon, Bridge, Bow, Fish, first half of Chest Stretch.

Low backache, Lumbago, Sciatica, Prolapsed intervertebral Disc
See the text, as degree of chronicity is important. Rabbit, Hare, Caterpillar and spinal flexion are wholly good. Posterior back stretches where lesion is chronic, also Coil, Pose of Child, mildly extending postures for early disc lesions, that is Bridge, Camel, Cat.

Postures to avoid with given disabilities

Cardiac and High Blood Pressure	avoid inverted postures
Eye and Ear Troubles	avoid inverted postures
Cervical Disc	avoid backward extension of head
Arthritis of Knees and Hips	avoid any forcing of knees to floor level

Severe prolapsed disc   avoid hyperextension of
                                      spine, never raise both legs
                                      off the ground together in
                                      any posture attempted.

Special Difficulties and Dangers

Osteoporosis is the biggest danger. If generalised osteoporosis
is known to be present, then everything must be done very
cautiously. Movements must be minimal and should involve
the *whole* spine, or *whole* limb, i.e. very gentle slow stretching
and relaxing. Rolling might be possible. Anything more
localised has to be introduced with great care.

Osteoarthritis, Rheumatoid Arthritis: The range of movements carried out in athritic joints should be increased only
very gradually, as circulation to the joints improves, and pain
lessens. An osteo-arthritic person can work through a mild
amount of pain, and will benefit; a person with rheumatoid
arthritis should not do this — he will come to harm.

10: Meditation

The yoga concept of meditation is that it is an approach through the mind to higher states of consciousness. By-products of meditation are contentment, happiness, peace of mind and tranquillity, alongside a knowledge of oneself that leads to a knowledge of life. The awareness that comes from meditation can and should be taken into other areas of life. The approach has to be one of effortless effort, and the ability to concentrate, developed through the exercises, overflows into every area.

The most important thing is not to try to solve outside problems, but to taste the present mood of peace, joy, happiness, flowing inside.

The meditations given here are all quite safe to do — they will not lead to any undesirable effect, such as overstimulated emotions or hallucinations. They are very elementary. Some of them, for example the meditation on the third eye, the sensation, the sound can also be starting points for more advanced meditation, which should only be embarked on with an experienced teacher. If the pupil is ready, the teacher will come. Meditation of that kind is not done at the end of a yoga practice session, but is something entirely of its own, to which increasing time has to be given, entirely separate from practical yoga sessions. *It is beyond the scope of this book.*

Here we are concerned only with some very simple meditative procedures, linked with the relaxation that should follow every session. However, the observed physiological effects of meditation proper — that is the slowing of the breathing rate, and rate of heartbeat, the drop in oxygen consumption, fall in metabolic rate — all take place. These result in a fall in blood pressure, and an increase in the slow alpha brain waves. These effects are just the opposite of the fight/flight reactions that accompany tension and anxiety. The way to combat stress is to direct the individual 'within' his own being, that is, to let him experience 'contact with himself'.

Some General Principles

Except when following immediately on a practice session (when it is practised lying down), meditation is best carried out sitting on the floor — there is something very healing about contact with Mother Earth. What is necessary is a straight spine and a firm solid base. The traditional Lotus posture is not for many Westerners — and certainly not for most of those with physical disabilities (except for one or two of the spastic or post-polio pupils for whom it may be quite effortless!) and indeed in this book, it has not been described. While being firmly based, the posture must be one in which it is possible to stay still for a considerable stretch of time.

The simple cross legged posture is perhaps the most suitable. If the knees come very high when the pupil is seated on the floor, then a pillow placed just under the buttocks, raising them off the floor, helps to bring the knees down and stabilise the posture; the feet should be as close to the groin as possible, the spine straight, the eyes closed, the backs of the hands resting on the knees, and the first finger and thumb of each hand touching.

Hero pose: Sitting back on or between the heels is more comfortable for some people, again with straight spine, and eyes closed, hands loosely resting on the thighs, with the first finger and thumb of each hand touching.

However, many people with physical disability will be quite unable to reach either of these two postures. If the whole session has been spent on the floor and is to be followed immediately by a form of simple meditation combined with relaxation, the most suitable arrangement is for the pupil to adopt any position on the floor in which he can be at ease and still for quite a time. This may be flat on the back — possibly with a support under the middle of the spine, — or even rolled on to one side, but still keeping the spine straight.

People who do their yoga sessions in wheelchairs or seated in ordinary chairs, and those who work on the floor but can in no way stay comfortably in any position there for as long as half an hour, should sit in chairs for meditation, the same rule applying — that is, straight spine and comfortable position. It is also necessary for the feet to be firmly planted on a solid surface, preferably straight.

Stillness is important, but regular practice at postures

develops a great deal of body control which ultimately shows as an ability to stay still. No one however should endure agonies of discomfort — the student should be told that if he gets uncomfortable he should shift gently until confortable again.

Breathing practice, at the beginning of yoga sessions, will have brought a degree of breath control and this in turn produces a calm mind. Slow relaxed breathing, with emphasis on the outbreath, the breath being allowed in gently as the body demands, results in a mind already calmed, with tension much reduced. This is the starting point for meditation. (*See below*, page 165)

From this starting point, awareness is developed, the essential self coming into its own as the mind is quietened down. The most natural method of all is that of 'awareness of the breath'. The pupil watches the breath, all the way in and all the way out. At the same time he must be aware of the body — the sensations of pain, discomfort, stiffness, itch. He may be able to relax through these, if not then he must scratch, move, shake — and restart, at the same time telling his mind to relax, and quietly returning to a concentration on the breath.

Later he turns to *observing* the thinking process, that is, to not becoming *part of* the thinking process, but becoming *aware* of it, being an *observer*. Most of the time we are all thinking endlessly about something or other, trapped within our own mind's workings! In meditation, the pupil just watches the ideas stream by, not interfering with them, not trying to stop them, explain them, or argue with them — just *observing*. When actual thinking stops, observing is what is left. This detached looking within is the most important part of meditation, for by means of it there is an approach to higher states of consciousness. These in their turn bring an understanding, an *awareness*, of the universe in which we live that is far beyond any mental concept of it that we might make. Furthermore the by-products of such an awareness are peace of mind, joy, understanding, happiness, and an unassailable tranquility, combined with a very deep and real knowledge of oneself.

Simple Meditations for beginners

The five simple examples of beginners' meditations that follow, which can be combined with the final relaxation of a yoga session, all make use of the sensation of movement, married up with the breath. The meditations present no problems. Even students who are mentally handicapped thoroughly enjoy them. In *every instance* the preliminaries are the same: 1) Unless following a yoga session, a suitable time of day must be chosen—early on is very good, as this is before too many outside problems and pressures have weighed in on the mind. 2) Too much light is to be avoided—it can be a distraction, concentration seems easier in more obscure lighting. 3) The position must be comfortable, one in which it is possible to stay still for half an hour. 4) Spine straight, not stiff. 5) Eyes closed. 6) Body energy circles complete—that is, thumb and first finger touching.

First check that there is no tension, that every part of the body is relaxed (see Relaxation, Chapter Three). This should be checked from head to foot—it is very important.

Second, pay attention to the breath—watch it coming in and going out, very gently, very quietly, and gradually getting a little slower. With breathing in, the abdomen rises, with breathing out it falls. The outbreath is a little longer than the inbreath, and is the more positive movement of the two. The inbreath just comes of its own accord, following a little pause after the outbreath. (Some of the phrases in the example below are used specifically because people with a physical handicap are envisaged.)

1) *The Cloud* (after preliminaries as listed above).
The voice of the leader should be quiet and calm, conducive of tranquility.

Now . . . you are lying on a cloud . . . a soft white cloud . . . and you have no stiffness and no discomfort . . . all you are aware of is softness . . . and warmth . . . and drifting . . . very slow, and very peaceful . . .

And gradually you can marry up the drifting movement with your breathing . . . as you breathe slowly out, the cloud drifts along . . . as you breathe in, the cloud gently stops—then it starts drifting once more as you breathe out, carrying on through the pause until you breathe in once more.

So you are just drifting . . . and stopping . . . and drifting . . . and stopping . . . and all you are aware of is the softness of the cloud round you, the warmth and comfort, and the oh so gentle movement . . . softness . . . warmth . . . and comfort . . . and gentle, gentle movement. Gentle movement . . .

Pause—In the early stages, the space of silent time in which there is no vocal direction is as little as two minutes, later this may be extended to three, five or whatever is most suitable for the group.

In your mind, let go of the movement . . . very gently . . .

Now quietly take your mind away from observing the breath . . .

Move your fingers, or your toes.

Move your head gently from side to side, so as to break the thread of inner concentration.

Then when you feel ready to, open your eyes. Taking a big action breath, stretch the whole body, arms and legs and head as widely as possible, screw the eyes up tight, re-open them and relax, then stretch.

Take a further big action breath and repeat the stretch.

Then when you feel you can—sit up (*if lying down*).

Try to carry away with you into the daily round some aware-ness—this is me, breathing deeply, this is me getting up, this is me putting on my shoes ready for activity. Hold on to the inner peace—turn back to survey it at intervals.

2) *The Canoe* (after the preparations as above).

Now you are lying on your back in a canoe, and it is very soft and very comfortable, just made to fit your shape . . . and you have no discomfort, no pain, no stiffness . . .

And the sun is shining, and the sky is blue, and the canoe is just drifting along . . . down a stream . . . And there is a little breeze just enough to keep the canoe moving . . . and you can hear the sound of trickling water . . . You can trail the fingers of one hand in the water, and feel the coldness of the water . . . on your fingertips.

And up above you can see the blue sky, through the branches of trees criss-crossing above you . . . And all you can feel is the warmth, and the comfort and the softness, and the cool of the water on the fingers of one hand . . .

And the movement of the canoe, just drifting gently forward—gently forward . . . just drifting . . .

And you can marry up the drifting of the canoe with your own breathing—as you breathe out it drifts gently forward, forward . . . and then after a pause, as you breathe in, the canoe slows up, or even stops . . .

With each outbreath, it drifts further and further forward . . . further and further forward . . . slowly drifting . . . and there is no ache, no stiffness . . .

And all you are conscious of is warmth, and comfort, and the cool water . . . and the oh so gentle movement . . . breathing out as the canoe drifts . . . out as the canoe drifts . . .

(Empty space of time. Then coming out of meditation—as in 1).

3) *The Swing* (after the preparations listed above).

Now you are sitting on a swing, very comfortably . . . all cushioned, and just shaped to fit around you—and you have no discomfort and no stiffness, no ache or pain of any kind . . .

And the sun is shining and the air is warm, and the swing is just gently moving backward and forward . . . backward and forward . . .

And all you can feel is warmth, and comfort, softness all round you . . . and gentle movement—backward and forward, backward and forward . . .

And you find you can marry up the gentle swinging movement with the movement of the breath . . . as you breathe out the swing moves forward, and as you breathe in, it moves back . . .

And moving forward is much longer and slower than moving back, which is really a very small movement . . .

And it is just backwards and forwards . . . slightly backwards and a long way forwards . . . and a very little backwards . . . and a long slow forwards . . . with no pain, no stiffness, and no discomfort.

And you are just conscious of warmth, and ease, and gentle movement—forward with the breath . . . forward with the breath . . .

(Empty space of time, then coming out of meditation as in 1).

4) *Over the Net* (after the preliminaries as listed above).

You are a small round ball, light and smooth . . . and you are being gently pushed over a net . . . from one side to the other . . .

Up and over—ever so gently; and then on the other side there is a hand ever so gently pushing you back again—up—and over—and down.

Then the first hand pushes you over again—up—and over . . . and then down on the second side . . . where the second hand reaches out and sends you back again, ever so gently—up and over . . . and down . . .

And all you feel is the gentle touch, and the slow movement up into the air, and over and down . . .

And you can marry the movement into your breathing —out as you go over and down and down . . .

And in as you go up—and going down is much further than going up . . . and goes on longer . . .

Gently up . . . then over and down and down—very slowly, very gently—backwards and forwards . . . from one side to the other . . .

Up . . . and over and down and down . . .

(Empty space of time, then coming out of meditation as in 1)

5) *The leaf in the wind* (after the preliminaries listed above).

You are like a small crumpled leaf, with no weight and no stiffness, just drifting before the wind . . . And the wind blows in little puffs . . . and it puffs you to the right . . . and then to the left . . . a little way up into the air . . . then you drop a little way down . . .

And the wind puffs again . . . and you go a little to the right . . . and a little to the left . . .

A little way up . . . then you drop a little way down . . . Then the wind blows a little less . . . and a little less . . . and so you move a little less to the right . . . a little less to the left . . . and a little bit less up . . . so you drop a little lower down . . .

And the puff of the wind gradually gets less and less . . . so you drop a little further down . . . and a little further down . . . and further down . . .

Until gently you drift to the ground . . . and you are so soft, so crumpled, that you just take the shape of the ground . . .

and yield into it . . .

And spread . . . and yield . . . into the ground—with no shape, no stiffness . . . just becoming part of the ground . . . given to the ground . . . into the ground . . .

(Empty space of time, then coming out of meditation as in 1)

A further Series of Meditations that can be tried when the previous five present no problems, and when the 'empty' period can be as long as five minutes. These five might be tried out in time given over to meditation only, i.e. with no posture work, if preferred, and if the pupils are keen.

The first step is to work on the ability to concentrate wholly at one point—that is 'one-pointedness', using the imagination as well, so as to deepen the awareness in every form of sensation.

1) *My name* (after the preliminaries as listed above)

Just in front of you there is a blackboard, square and shiny; underneath are pieces of coloured chalk. Pick up whatever colour you like and, standing in front of the board, close to it, begin to write your own name—

Write it slowly, with long flowing curves—as if in one continuous letter. Focus your attention totally on the end of the chalk just where it touches the board . . .

Focus every scrap of your attention on that meeting of chalk and board, where the point of the writing is; follow every curving movement of the chalk . . . exactly as it is made . . .

Be careful not to move your head as the chalk moves—it is just the attention that moves—your full attention totally concentrated on the tip of the chalk . . .

Write in long flowing curves . . . follow the tip of the chalk with your attention . . .

Take your time . . . let the chalk move slowly . . . All your attention totally focussed on the point of the chalk . . . Take your time . . .

When you have completely finished the flowing curves of your name, put a full stop . . . move away from the board little by little—

Keep your eyes and attention fully focussed on your writing.

Bit by bit as you move back you see more and more of what you have written . . .

Keep your gaze fixed on the writing . . .

Move very slowly back . . .

Stop when you have the whole name in your gaze . . . and look steadily at the whole name, and the board . . . *(Pause)* Gently and slowly move back towards the board—little by little—keep your full attention focussed on the writing . . . you see less and less of it . . .

Go on moving forward with the name getting smaller and smaller . . . until there is only one small point within your sight . . .

Keep your gaze fixed on this one point—watch it getting fainter and fainter . . . and fainter—till finally it goes right away . . . and there is nothing to be seen . . . just nothing . . . nothing . . .

(Empty space of time. Then come out of meditation exactly as in the first series).

2) *Relaxation sensation*

Perform this lying down comfortably, preferably in the floor posture, and without a pillow. This position may be thoroughly uncomfortable in some forms of physical disability: so a comfortable one must be found, and the text below altered accordingly! (The meditator is not meant to fall asleep during this!). It is as well to have a rug over the body as in relaxation, and to remain perfectly still with the eyes closed—stillness is perhaps more important in this than in other methods.

Make sure you are perfectly comfortable, and now relax . . . let the whole body go limp . . .

Lift your head an inch or two off the ground, then let it go back, relaxed to the neck . . .

Lift your shoulders off the ground—and put them back relaxed and loosened . . .

Lift the arms . . . tensing the elbows, wrists and the fingers—then let them all relax on to the floor . . .

Tighten the muscles of the chest on an inbreath, let them all relax on an outbreath . . .

Tighten all the tummy muscles . . . let them all relax . . .

Tighten the thighs . . .

The knees . . .

Ankles, feet, toes . . . lifting the heels off the ground . . .

Sink down into the ground, relax, relax . . .

Be aware of the whole of yourself lying on the floor . . . the whole body —

Now concentrate all your attention on:

the right heel touching the floor . . . the exact spot

then the left heel touching the floor . . . the exact spot

then the right calf touching the floor . . . the exact spot

and the left calf touching the floor . . . the exact spot

then the right thigh touching the floor . . . the exact spot

and the left thigh touching the floor . . . the exact spot

and the right buttock touching the floor . . . the exact spot

and the left buttock touching the floor . . . the exact spot

Next the small of the back touching the floor . . . the exact spot

and from the waist upwards, where it touches the floor

then the right shoulder blade, where it touches the floor

and the left shoulder blade where it touches the floor

Next all the fingers of the right hand where they touch the floor

and all the fingers of the left hand where they touch the floor

and the right hand itself where it touches the floor

and the left hand itself where it touches the floor

Next the right elbow where it touches the floor

and the left elbow where it touches the floor

Now the top of the right arm where it touches the floor

and the top of the left arm where it touches the floor

Now the back of the neck where it touches the floor

and the back of the head where it touches the floor

Now once again feel the sensation of the whole body touching the floor at the same time . . . the floor and the body, the floor and the body.

Feel the total strength of this area of contact . . . the floor and the body — concentrate your full attention on this — the floor and the body . . . the floor and the body . . .

(Empty space of time coming out as in series one)

3) *Sound — and obliteration of sound* (after the preliminaries as in series one, but omitting the attention to the breath)

Start with five rounds of alternate nostril breathing (see Chapter Four).

Follow with seven 'bee' breaths (See Chapter Four).

Become 'aware' of sound . . . aware of sound . . . of sound

Be aware of every sound you can hear, identify it . . .

Pick out the sounds one by one . . . identifying each one . . . the loudest first . . .

The aeroplane going over . . . the traffic, car coming up the road . . . be aware of sound . . .

The dog barking . . . Footsteps overhead . . .

The distant hum of the boiler underlying everything . . .

The clock ticking . . . be aware of every sound—all sound

Slight movement . . . rustle of clothes around you . . .

(then proceed with either variation one, or two).

VARIATION ONE

Your neighbour breathing . . . Your own breathing . . .

(Use the heart beat if preferred).

Focus all your attention on the breath (or heart beat) . . . You know what every other sound is—let it flow over you—just be aware of the breath (or heartbeat)—your own breath, (or heartbeat), nothing else but your own breath (or heartbeat) . . . gently out . . . pause—no definite in breath, let the air just 'trickle' in as need be . . .

Breath going out . . .

Breath going out . . .

(Empty space of time—coming out of meditation as in series one)

VARIATION TWO

Now you have heard and identified every sound . . . listen to the silence . . .

You can still hear the sounds . . . pay no attention to them . . . hear them and let them go . . . now listen to the silence within you . . .

The silence you can find within you . . .

Listen . . . is there any inner sound in that silence . . .

Just listen—to any sound there is welling up in the silence within you

Inner silence . . . inner silence . . . inner sound . . . inner sound . . . inner sound

(Empty space of time . . . coming out of meditation as in series one)

4) *Meditation with the help of a Mantra* After the usual preliminaries as in series one.

Take your mantra — 'peace' . . . concentrate all your attention on this . . . 'peace' . . . repeat it in your mind slowly and lingeringly . . . 'peace' . . . 'peace' . . .

Draw the word gently into yourself — take it in through the space that lies between your two eyes . . . 'peace' . . . 'peace' . . . through the space between the eyes . . . take 'peace' right down inside yourself . . . 'peace' . . . 'peace'.

With each breath *out* . . . draw your mantra 'peace' further down into yourself — very slowly, very gently . . . 'peace' . . . 'peace' . . . draw it down within . . . fold it deep within you . . . 'peace' — right down into the depths of your being . . . 'peace' . . . Hold it there . . . 'peace' . . . fold it into yourself . . . 'peace' . . . 'peace' . . .
(Empty space of time . . . then coming out of meditation as in series one)

There are many suitable mantras — love, joy, God is, I am, God; for the Christian — Father, Lord Jesus Christ; be still, tranquillity, bliss, friends: one of the most satisfactory is OM — a syllable meaning God, much used in chanting. Often the use of a Mantra is combined with the use of a Mala, in which a string of beads, usually 108 in number, moving one bead for each repetition, rather like a rosary is used.

5) *Seeing the Third Eye* (after the preliminaries as in series one)
Chant OM *seven times, holding the* MMM *each time till breathing out finishes but with no strain.*
Gently focus your attention on the space between the eyebrows — keep relaxed — only the attention is focussed.

You may lick your finger and touch the spot — make sure the attention is fixed where you have placed the dot . . .

See a small star where you finger touched and made the dot . . .

Concentrate on this star — watch it — keep relaxed in yourself but watch the star . . .

Imagine a small seed inside . . . a coloured seed — pink or green, blurred in outline . . . watch it — without strain . . . watch the seed . . . watch it glowing . . . becoming clearer . . . and clearer . . .

Keep your attention focussed between the eyebrows . . .
watch the seed as it glows . . . the star is a glowing seed . . .
The only sensation you have is an awareness of this seed — the
seed between the eyebrows — the seed . . . glowing — the
glowing seed . . .

*(Empty space of time — coming out of meditation as in series
one).*

6 a) *Candle Flame* (real — that is, with an actual candle on the
floor — hence sitting up is necessary. After the preliminaries as
in series one).

Fix the gaze — without any strain — on the tip of the candle
in front of you . . .

Watch the tip of the flame as it flickers . . .

Try to avoid blinking — close the eyes as soon as they feel any
strain — then open them again gently . . .

Watch the tip of the flame . . . watch the flame and the
flicker . . . close the eyes . . . see the colour that appears in
the centre between the eyebrows . . . appearing . . . dis-
appearing . . . When the colour has gone, open the eyes again
and look at the tip of the candle flame, gently ,with no
tension . . . relax . . . but focus . . . on the tip . . .

Now close the eyes . . . watch for the colours . . . watch the
colours that may appear . . . do not follow them with the eyes
if they move . . . quietly watch the centre between the
eyes . . . quietly return to the candle with eyes open when the
colours go . . . and back again to the third eye . . . and back
to the candle tip . . . the colours . . . the candle . . .
colours . . . candle . . .

*(Empty space of time. Coming out of meditation as in series
one).*

6 b) *Candle Flame* (imaginary, after preliminaries as in series
one).

In front of you, you can see a candle flame flickering — a
gold flame curling into a brownish black tip with smoke . . .
there is a bluish edge . . .

The wick has a pool of candle grease around it . . . below
this is the candle — thick or thin, smooth or ridged, or with a
pattern, or picture . . .

What colour is it — red — blue — green — yellow — mauve

—brown—cream—move the eyes to the base of the candle . . . see it complete . . . candle and flame . . . see the whole candle, colour, texture, shape . . . Look further down still . . . beneath the candle is a candlestick . . . wood . . . or glass . . . or brass . . . or iron . . . or silver . . . or pottery . . .

It has a colour too . . . and a shape . . . a design . . .

And a definite size . . . see the whole candle with the candlestick . . .

Look further down still, . . . and it is standing on a small stool or table . . . the table has three or four legs . . . it is wooden . . . plain or ornate . . . polished or painted . . .

Now you see the whole picture—candle flame . . . candle . . . candle stick . . . support . . . see all colours, materials, textures . . . shapes . . . sizes . . .

Now quietly take your gaze back up . . . the supporting table or stool . . . the candle stick—notice the material, the shape, the colour . . . The candle itself . . . notice the shape—fat/thin—smooth/ridged, any pattern, picture . . . the colour . . .

Now the flame with its flickering tip . . . Focus on the flickering—tip—no tension—very gentle—without straining . . .

The flickering tip of the candle . . . you are aware of what else is there by but you do not see it—only the tip, flickering . . . flickering . . .

(Empty space of time—coming out of meditation as in series one).

7) *The Tunnel* (after preliminaries)

You are in a dark tunnel, moving through it—with no difficulty . . . just flowing . . . no stiffness . . . gently flowing . . .

The tunnel is quite dark, the walls are black . . . at the very end you can see a pinpoint of light . . .

Fix your eyes on the light . . . without strain—just move . . . flow . . . effortlessly towards it . . .

As you move gently along, with no effort . . . the little pinpoint of light gradually gets bigger . . . and less faint . . .

It is quite a round hole of light . . . getting bigger . . . As you get nearer and nearer so it begins to reflect off the walls . . . now the walls are getting lighter . . . and lighter . . .

And the light at the end is bigger — and bigger . . . and brighter and brighter . . .

And you get closer . . . and closer to it . . . and closer . . . And you move out into bright light and warmth . . . fully out into light and warmth . . . light and warmth . . .

(Minute or two in silence)

Then . . . Embrace the light and warmth and fold them inside you . . . deep inside you . . . quietly begin to move backwards into the tunnel . . .

Moving backwards . . . gently . . . and effortlessly . . .

Backwards . . . and as you go the light at the end of the tunnel gets smaller . . . and fainter . . . and it is no longer thrown up on the walls . . . the walls become darker and darker . . .

And the light at the end is smaller . . . and fainter and smaller . . . and fainter . . .

Until there is nothing . . . only dark . . . but you are full of light and warmth . . . hold them folded inside yourself . . . light and warmth . . . light and warmth . . . deep inside you . . .

(Empty space of time . . . coming out of meditation as in series one).

The Use of a Yantra

Meditation can be practised with the use of a Yantra — that is a geometric design, on the wall. The preparation is as usual, and then the gaze is fixed without tension on the design, and the mind is left empty, the gaze just accepting the 'movement' in the design. It is better not to think, but to close the eyes at any feeling of strain, then quietly reopen them. Yantras can be in black and white, or coloured. Children get great joy out of designing their own. Much of the abstract work that physically handicapped people with little hand control, or perhaps painting with a brush in the mouth, do in their art classes, or the designs the elderly may do if they take to art late in life, can be used to good effect.

A Yantra is particularly useful for those who find it difficult to concentrate on the spoken word.

To recapitulate: the first series in this chapter is very useful used at the end of a practical session; the second series, though longer, can be used in the same way, or in separate sessions. All are totally safe and will produce no undesirable effects. For use with yourself, record them on to a cassette slowly and quietly, using a very tranquil voice, and plenty of pause.

More advanced meditation must be taught by an experienced teacher.

Appendix I

What is Yoga?

This appendix claims no more than to give a few pointers towards answering that question, giving some very slight idea of the art and science of yoga, as well as defining a few yoga expressions to be found in the text.

The word 'yoga' stems from a Sanskrit word having many shades of meaning; basically it means 'union', and is often taken to mean the integration of body, mind and spirit into one harmonious whole. Ultimately it means the union of the personal spirit with the Divine Spirit — whether this be called God, the one Being, the Absolute, or some other name. Consequently the true aim of yoga is spiritual, although it is not itself a religion. Adherents to all religions practise yoga, which cannot conflict with their religious beliefs, since all religions teach the Omnipotence, the Omnipresence of 'One' bringing order into the universe.

The yoga tenet is that God is Omnipresent — a universal principle to be found in everyone and everything. Practising yoga, the individual gets to know his real self, and to find the 'God within'; knowing himself, his line of thought becomes truly positive; finding God, he is full of compassion.

Hatha Yoga
Some very elementary principles and practices of Hatha yoga are described in this book. This yoga covers the physical aspect, it is yoga of postures. Yoga to many in the Western world means just that — a system of exercises producing health and energy. In reality Hatha yoga prepares the way for the search for God, since it helps the practitioner to acquire control of mind and body. It is closely linked with his conduct of his own life, for he recognises — and shows by his life style that he recognises — the fact that the material aspect of life is not the only one. Since the body is the temple of the spirit, the Hatha yoga practitioner 'cares' for it, so that it may be a fitting temple, and furthermore a cogent means whereby the spirit is expressed. There are many other 'yogas' — see below for a very few.

Raja Yoga and other Yogas
One of the many other forms of yoga, Raja yoga is termed the king of yogas, the yoga of the intellect, in which the seeker makes use of

the intellect to reach his goal, and acquire mastery over inner powers. Then there is Gnana yoga—the yoga of knowledge, of wisdom, in which the proper value and use is attached to all things. In Gnana yoga, knowledge has to be felt, not just known, and the practitioner is always seeking deeper knowledge of the life force that exists in everything, even inanimate objects. Karma yoga is the yoga of action, of work done for one's fellows, without expectation of reward, selfless work for the benefit of others, done in a spirit of detachment—unworried over the results. Bhakti yoga is the yoga of devotion to what is Divine, to Goodness in all things. It calls for self-surrender, a devotion that stems from the appreciation of the Good. It is a love of that which is wholly good—for the reason of its Goodness. Kriya yoga has three sections— the organisation of the body, the development of the mind, and attention to spiritual progress. Hatha yoga, the yoga of postures has to do with the first section, along with certain practices of purification called Kriyas. The essence of the second section is study—as for example, the study of yoga itself ; the practice of meditation leads eventually to the awareness of Divinity, which is the goal of section three.

Some aids to the practice of Yoga
Mantra (the yoga of sound):

Use is made of sound to help the individual in meditation along the spiritual path, by the repetition of a whole phrase, a single word, or single sound. (In Sanskrit the syllable *man* means 'to think', and *tra* means 'means of' hence a *mantra* is a 'means of thinking'.)

AUM—known as the Sacred Syllable, because it refers to the Divine Essence—is perhaps the commonest. When chanted it is pronounced OME, but may be pronounced as three syllables, sustained and vibrating—AW—OO—MMMM. It is found that chanting this—slowly, holding the sound till the breath gives out, then repeating with a fresh intake of breath, uplifts the whole being. Try it! Chanting a mantra gives an inner mental vibration, besides the actual echoing physical resonance heard extensively. Can you feel it?

A famous Tibetan mantra is AUM MARE PADME HUM— hail to the jewel in the lotus, AUM SHANTI SHANTI is hail, peace, peace. Some yoga teachers like to precede their classes chanting AUM together, and finish with SHANTI, SHANTI. Christians often prefer as mantras, words and phrases like 'God is', 'Love', 'Be still', 'Christ have mercy'. See Chapter Ten, Meditation, Series Two, number 4.

Mala.

This is a string of 108 beads, used as an aid to saying, or silently repeating, the mantra, by passing the fingers on to the next bead after each repetition. (A mala may be half the number of beads—54, or double — 216). It is usually made of wood, perhaps of shells or seeds (something of life) and may be worn or carried — carried obviously for use. The 108 beads are joined, in a circle, by means of a different bead which also carries a tuft of hair. On feeling this, the fingers turn round and go back again, never actually crossing the middle bead. Using a mala is termed Japa yoga.

Yantra Yoga. The Yoga of design.

(Mandala is the word often used for these designs — though really this means simply a circle.) Geometrical designs are used to help in spiritual development — as is the mantra previously described. A yantra may be said to be a concept of divinity, it is often a series of interlaced triangles; or petal shapes — representing the petals of the lotus flower — may also be used. Man has his roots on earth, as the lotus has its roots in the mud at the bottom of the river; man must ever reach upwards towards the divine, as the lotus blooms on breaking the surface of the water.

A few definitions that may help

Abdominal lock ⎫
Anal lock ⎭ . . . . See under Bandha.

Bandha A chaining or fettering. The word describes a posture in which certain organs or parts of the body are contracted. When the chin rests in the sternal notch at the top of the breast bone and the neck and throat are contracted (*the chin lock*), then the flow of blood and prana to heart, scalp, brain and thyroid is regulated. It occurs in the shoulder stand, and is also an essential factor in many pranayamic practices. When the abdominal muscles are pulled forcefully back towards the spine, manipulating the diaphragm upwards, this is termed *the abdominal lock*. It is performed at the end of exhalation, and in the pause between that and further inhalation, but must never be performed between inhalation and exhalation. It exercises the diaphragm and abdominal muscles, compresses the abdominal organs and massages the heart muscle. When the perianal muscles are contracted and the anus tightened, pulling all the lower abdominal area up and backwards towards the spine, this is termed the *anal lock*.

Chakra Psychic centres, of which there are six principal ones, which are to be found at the base of the spine, the sacral area, the solar plexus, the heart, the throat and the brow. Psychic energy rises up the spine to the top of the head, passing from chakra to chakra to a seventh on the top of the head, the 'thousand petalled lotus'.

Guru A spiritual guide. The word *Gu* means darknesss — the guru brings light into the darkness, *ru* meaning light.

Kundalini A coiled female serpent. It stands for the cosmic energy lying dormant at the base of the spine, and rising through the chakras (q.v.) to the thousand petalled lotus in the head, putting the individual in union with the Universal Soul.

Lotus posture—padmasana Sitting in the lotus posture is the ideal posture for meditation, but is possible to few of us Westerners, accustomed as we are to sitting on chairs from childhood. You will not find it described in the chapters on postures, but a few spastic people, and many people who have had polio with residual flaccid paralysis, go into it with ease and sit in it of choice for comfort! It is achieved as follows:

Sit on the floor with legs stretched straight out;
Bend the right leg, hold the foot with both hands and place it at the very top of the left thigh, so that the right heel is near the umbilicus;
Bend the left leg, hold the foot with both hands and place it over the right leg at the top of the right thigh, so that the left heel is near the navel;
The soles of both feet are turned upwards;
Keep the spine erect, place the right hand on the right knee, the left hand on the left knee, palms uppermost, with the forefingers and thumbs bent and touching.

Prana Universal energy and the source of all energy, present everywhere and in everything; prana is mostly absorbed with the breath, and stored when the breath is held, stored mainly in the solar plexus. Prana is also taken in with food and drink. Prana is manifested in practical action, in creative art and in intellectual activity. It behaves like some kind of electricity. Pranayama yoga deals with the intake and the control of prana.

Rishi A wise man, a sage.

The Third Eye A psychic spot between the eyebrows. At first human beings had only one eye, so it is said, placed in the middle of the forehead. This eye disappeared as the two-eye arrangement evolved, enabling man to see at a much wider angle. The third eye was sensitive to vibrations, it now lies dormant but can be awakened. Thoughts appear to stream out from the third eye centre, and if the individual focusses all his attention on the area he can see visions. For many people it comes naturally to turn eyes and attention upwards towards the third eye when concentrating.

Yogi Man who practises yoga.

Yogini Woman who practises yoga.

A little bit about Yogic 'writings'.

Sanskrit The ancient language of India in which the Bhagavad Gita, the Sutras of Patanjali and the Upanishads are written.
Yoga postures have Sanskrit names—see Appendix III.
Sanskrit has not been used in the text.

Bhagavad Gita Often spoken of simply as the Gita. This is a collection of sacred dialogues between a warrior Arjuna and his charioteer Krishna, written about 500 BC and first translated into English in 1785. The dialogues portray the struggle of the human soul towards a vision of God in all things and all things in God. The yoga of the Gita is the yoga of love.

The aphorisms or sutras of Patanjali Those who have heard anything about the underlying philosophy of yoga will have heard of Patanjali, who coordinated the yoga system of philosophy into 185 aphorisms (short sayings) more than 2,000 years ago. These aphorisms or sutras, classifying the eight limbs or stages of yoga with their Sanskrit names, are as follows:

1. *Yama* Conduct towards others—non-injury, truthfulness, non-theft, self-discipline, non-greed!

2. *Nyama* Conduct towards oneself—cleanliness, contentment, austerity, self-study, attentiveness to God.

3. *Hatha yoga* The yoga of postures. *Ha* meaning sun, *tha* meaning moon.

4. *Pranayama* Breath control, including the control of the intake and storing of the vital energy, cosmic energy, prana.

5. *Pratyahara* Control of the senses resulting in one-pointedness of mind.

6. *Dharana* Concentration on one thing to the exclusion of all else, fixing the mind on a target and not letting it wander. The target may be tangible or abstract—a candle flame, the idea of love.

7. *Dhyana* Meditation. The extension of concentration, mental effort applied to a chosen object or topic: it is a spiritual process, and the individual lets intruding thoughts come and go, and returns calmly to his subject.

8. *Samadhi* The highest form of Union with the Divine—the supreme goal. Contemplation—described by Suzuki as 'quiet tranquil equilibrium such as that of the ocean on a quiet night reflecting the stars when there are no waves stirring.'

Upanishads These writings are the philosophical part of the Vedas, which are the most ancient sacred literature of the Hindus. This is a literature dealing with the nature of man, the nature of the universe, the union of the individual soul with the Universal soul.

Appendix II

Anatomical, Physiological, Medical Terms

These definitions are not complete, they serve only to clarify the text. Consequently they are minimal, defining to the extent that the word has been used in this book and no more.

Abdomen The part of the trunk situated between the thorax and the pelvis (q.v.). It contains the stomach, small and large intestine, liver, gall bladder, spleen and pancreas. These constitute the abdominal viscera.

Abduction A drawing away, the action of a muscle that draws a limb away from another limb, or the midline of the body, e.g. the abductors of the legs separate the legs.

Achilles tendon See *Tendon*.

Adduction A drawing towards, the action of a muscle that draws a limb towards another limb, or the midline of the body, e.g. the adductors of the legs, if contracted, make it difficult for the legs to open.

Alpha Brain Waves Slow rhythmic oscillations of electric potential (roughly 10 per second) predominating during relaxation states, and seen when a tracing is taken of the brain functioning. Other waves predominate at other times.

Alveolus (pl. *alveoli*) An air cell in the lungs across the wall of which oxygen and carbon dioxide are interchanged. See *Respiration*.

Ankylosing Spondylitis (syn. Poker or Bamboo spine.) Disease in which the whole spine becomes rigid due to changes, similar to those of rheumatoid arthritis, occuring in the intervertebral joints.

Anus The end of the digestive tract, where the rectum discharges the faeces, (q.v.) from the body. It is under voluntary muscular control. The perianal muscles—that is the muscles round the anus, involved in the act of defaecation—are tightened in many of the 'locks'—see Appendix One, used in breath control.

Arteriosclerosis The term applied to a number of conditions in which there is thickening or hardening of the arteries, with loss of elasticity.

It can result from a number of factors—aging, faulty fat metabolism, high blood pressure, overweight, cigarette smoking, physical inactivity, inability to cope with stress. See *Cardiovascular System*.

Arthritis Inflammation of a joint, which may be acute or chronic. The commonest types are osteo—and rheumatoid. Osteoarthritis is a chronic disease involving mainly weight-bearing joints. The joint surface degenerates, resulting in pain and impairment of function. Rheumatoid arthritis is a chronic systematic disease with gross inflammatory changes in joints, mainly the smaller ones, resulting in pain and crippling deformities.

Asthma Paroxysmal difficulty in breathing, caused by spasm of the bronchial tubes or swelling of their lining, resulting in wheezing. The spasm inhibits breathing out—consequently breathing in is difficult, the lungs being full. Attacks are caused by infection or allergy, but fatigue, tension, emotion play a strong part in triggering off the paroxysms.

Ataxia Incoordination of muscular activity—particularly that of voluntary muscular movement e.g. walking. A reeling or staggering gait is described as ataxic.

Atheroma Fatty degeneration, thickening of the walls of arteries occurring in atherosclerosis, one form of arteriosclerosis (q.v.).

Athetosis The condition in which there are involuntary slow, irregular movements in arms, legs and head due to a lesion in the brain.

Athetoid—affected by athetosis.

Autonomic Nervous System See *Nervous System*.

Blood Pressure The pressure existing in large arteries due to the passage of blood through the artery. The systolic blood pressure is produced by the contraction of the heart, while the diastolic occurs in the relaxation phase between heartbeats. Blood pressure is measured against a column of mercury by means of a sphygomanometer, compressing the artery and then released until the heart sounds are just audible with a stethoscope. It is expressed in figures e.g. 120/70. The lower figure is the more significant. The upper figure is affected by excitement and emotion, etc. Blood pressure may be normal, high or low. Abnormal systolic is reckoned to be above 140 or below 100, and abnormal diastolic is reckoned to be above 100 or below 65. See *Cardiovascular system*.

Bronchitis Inflammation of the linings of the bronchial tubes; the disease may be acute or chronic, and is due to bacterial infection.

Bronchus (pl. *bronchi*) One of two large branches—passageways for air—off the windpipe, each leading to a lung and subdividing into smaller and ever smaller tubes—the bronchioles. See *Respiratory system*.

Buttocks (syn. bottom) Fleshy part of the body posterior to the hip joints. The buttocks are formed by large masses of muscles called the glutei.

Carbon Dioxide (CO_2) Colourless gas, waste product of the body metabolism, carried from the tissues by the red blood cells to the lungs, where it passes into the alveoli, hence into the bronchioles and subsequently out through mouth or nose. The level of carbon dioxide in the blood to a great extent controls the respiratory rate.

Carcinoma A new growth, malignant tumour, neoplasm, syn. cancer. These tumours invade surrounding tissues and give rise to secondaries elsewhere in the body, spreading both by means of circulating blood and lymphatics. Carcinoma may affect any organ or part of the body.

Cardiovascular System The circulatory system consisting of heart, and blood vessels—that is, arteries, arterioles, capillaries, venules and veins.

Cartilage (gristle) Connective tissue of various types—for example joining the ribs to the breast bone, covering joint surfaces, in the knee joint.

Central Nervous System CNS See *Nervous System*.

Cervical Pertaining to the neck e.g. cervical disc, cervical muscles, cervical vertebrae—see *Vertebra*.

Circulation of the blood The blood leaves the left ventricle of the heart, passing into the aorta, thence into first larger then smaller arteries, arterioles, all over the body, finally into the capillaries. Passing through the capillaries it is gathered into small venules, then veins gradually increasing in size until it is returned to the right side of the heart via the great veins. From the right side of the heart it is pumped into arteries taking it to the lungs, where the carbon dioxide carried by the red cells passes through the alveolar wall in exchange for oxygen. The newly oxygenated blood is then returned to the left side of the heart to recirculate.

Congenital Present at birth.

Diaphragm A strong muscle separating the abdominal from the thoracic cavity. It is convex upwards and contracts downwards on each inspiration, allowing the lower lobes of the lungs to expand downwards. On expiration it relaxes, elevating itself upwards again. The deeper the inspiration and expiration, the greater the range of diaphragmatic movement. The great blood vessels carrying blood to and from the heart, to and from the trunk and lower limbs, pass through the diaphragm, as does the oesophagus (q.v.).

Diaphragmatic Hernia Protrusion of the stomach upwards into the thoracic cavity through the hole in the diaphragm carrying the oesophagus (q.v.). It occurs when the hole becomes lax.

Digestive System The body system concerned with the digestion of food, comprising mouth, oesophagus (the tube between the mouth and the stomach), stomach, duodenum (the first part of the small intestine, leading out of the stomach), the small intestine, large intestine, rectum and anus. Digestion is the process whereby food is broken down mechanically and chemically and converted into forms usable by the body after absorption.

Disc See *Vertebra*.

Dorsal Appertaining to the back, or indicating a position towards the back as opposed to the front.

Dorsum Posterior surface of, as the dorsum or back of the hand; referring to the foot it means the upper surface.

Dysmenorrhoea Painful or difficult monthly periods in women. It may be primary or secondary. In primary dysmenorrhoea there is no underlying disease as cause. Secondary dysmenorrhoea may be due to congestion or inflammation in the pelvis (q.v.). It may start before the period and finish shortly after the period starts, or it may start some time after the period has started. In some cases it lasts throughout. Pain varies from mild to very severe.

Embryo The stage in development that comes between the second and eighth week of intra-uterine development.

Endocrine glands Glands without ducts, whose secretion is passed directly into the bloodstream or lymphatic system. Consequently the hormones they secrete produce their effects at some distance from the gland. Endocrine glands include the pituitary, thyroid, parathyroids, adrenal (suprarenal), the Islets of Langerhans—found in the pancreas, testes and ovaries. Some of the hormones affect the metabolism of the whole body e.g. thyroxin secreted by the thyroid. Dysfunction of endocrine glands results from either over or under secretion.

Epiglottis See *Glottis*.

Exercise Tolerance A measurement of the efficiency of the cardiac and respiratory systems. A measured amount of work is performed in relation to oxygen consumption and rise in rate of heartbeat. A simple home test is that of running on the spot for a given length of time, then seeing how long it takes for pulse and respiratory rate to return to normal — this should be less than two minutes.

Extension Movement pulling two ends further apart, the opposite of flexion. In spinal extension, the trunk bends backwards; in extension of the elbow, the arm straightens.

Faeces The waste products of digestion, the stools (consisting of food residue, bacteria, debris from the lining of the intestines, and mucus) discharged from the intestinal tract by way of the anus.

Flaccid A form of paralysis (q.v.).

Flexion Movement pulling two ends together, the opposite of extension. The arm is flexed if bent at the elbow, bringing the hand towards the shoulder; the trunk is flexed if the head and upper part of the body are bent over towards the feet.

Foetus The child in utero between the third month and birth.

Friedreich's ataxia An inherited degenerative disease of the central nervous system characterised by ataxia (q.v.), impairment of speech, and paralysis, particularly of the lower limbs. The disease may show in infancy, or start in adolescence.

Ganglion (pl. ganglia) Clumps of nerve tissue, consisting mainly of nerve cells bodies, but lying outside the brain and spinal cord. See *Nervous system.*

Glottis The two vocal cords and the space that lies between them, that is, part of the voice box or larynx (q.v.) by means of which sound is actually produced. The epiglottis is a little lid covering the glottis.

Hormone The secretion of the ductless glands, as for example thyroxin of the thyroid, insulin of the islets of Langerhans.

Hydrocephalus The accumulation of the protective fluid which bathes the brain and the spinal cord within the ventricles or air cavities of the brain. It results from faulty circulation of this fluid due to maldevelopment of the brain before birth. Unless the condition is relieved by surgery, the head gets larger and larger, and the brain cells are compressed by the excess fluid. Surgical treatment lies in inserting a valve enabling the fluid to circulate.

Hypertension See *Blood pressure* Condition where the blood pressure is higher than normal. There are many causes, among which thickening or hardening of the arteries is the commonest.

Ileal loop Diverting the urinary flow by transplanting the ureters into an isolated segment of small intestine, the other end of which opens on to the abdominal wall, where the urine is collected in a special bag. See *Renal system*.

Ileum Lower three-fifths of the small intestine running into the large intestine.

Infantile Paralysis (syn. anterior poliomyelitis — polio) An acute inflammatory infection of the cells of the central nervous system in the spinal cord. Due to a virus, it may be mild or severe. Since the virus destroys the nerve cells, it invades the muscles supplied by their nerve fibres, which atrophy cannot function. The paralysis produced is flaccid.

Intercostal muscles Muscles lying between the ribs — arising from the lower edge of one rib and inserted into the upper edge of the rib below. Together with the ribs, breastbone and spine, they form the walls of the thoracic cavity. Their function, working with the diaphragm, is to increase the size of the cavity, drawing the ribs upwards and outwards.

Intervertebral disc (syn. spinal disc) Fibrocartilaginous disc lying between the bodies of the spinal vertebrae, (the bones that make up the spine). See *Vertebra*.

Intervertebral joints The joint which occurs between the bones of the spinal column — the vertebrae (q.v.).

Joint The juncture between two bones. There are several types, classified according to the type of movement taking place between the two surfaces. Two common types are hinge joints, e.g. the knee, with movement in two directions only like a hinge, that is flexion and extension; and ball and socket joints, where the rounded end of one bone fits into a cavity in the other, e.g. the hip, where movements are flexion, extension, internal and external rotation (q.v.).

Lateral Pertaining to the side. Lateral flexion — bending to the side.

Latissimus dorsi A broad strong muscle covering a large part of the lower and middle back, arising from the bones of the spine and inserted into the upper part of the arm.

Larynx The voice box at the upper end of the trachea below the root of the tongue. It forms the prominent Adam's apple in the male.

Lesion An injury, wound, something wrong. A boil is a lesion of the skin, so is a rash.

Ligament Band of strong fibrous tissue attaching bones together, attaching muscle to bone, or forming a support for joints, e.g. the ligaments surrounding the shoulder joint or hip joint.

Lumbar region The loins. The areas on either side of the lumbar vertebrae (q.v.).

Lumbar spine The lower part of the spinal column; the fifth (and lowest) lumbar vertebra forms a joint with the sacrum.

Medulla Oblongata A thickened part of the spinal cord, found at the top just inside the skull, below the mid-brain. It contains the respiratory centre, from which the respiration is controlled — that part of the control which lies outside the voluntary control exercised by the individual.

Menstruation Discharge from the uterus (womb) of a bloody fluid occurring at intervals of roughly one month, during the child bearing period of a woman's life, approximately 13–52 years, but very variable.

Metabolism The sum total of all the physical and chemical changes that take place within the body.

Motor Neurone Disease A motor neuron consists of a nerve cell and its fibre carrying the impulse which will stimulate a muscle fibre to contract. In this disease the cell dies, the impulse cannot be conducted, and the muscle fibre ceases to function. The resultant disability depends upon what muscles are supplied by the affected nerve cells.

Muscular Dystrophy Wasting away of muscles. The term is applied to a number of diseases, some of them hereditary, in which this is the symptom. The resultant disability depends upon the function of the affected muscles. There are variations in age of onset, in the sex carrying the disease, the muscles affected and the rate of deterioration.

Multiple Sclerosis A progressive degenerating disease of the central nervous system with muscular weakness, leading to paralysis and tremor, also speech, sight and swallowing difficulties, all due to an impairment of motor impulses to muscles. A disease mainly of young adults, both sexes, often of sudden onset, characterised by exacerbation and remissions. Cause still unknown — not hereditary.

Nervous System There are two — the central nervous system and the autonomic nervous system.

The central nervous system (CNS) consists of the brain, spinal cord, nerve cells, nerve fibres and nerve endings that control voluntary activity. Cells are present in brain and cord. Fibres carry impulses from the cells to the various body tissues. They also carry information from end organs in the tissues back to the cord and brain.

The autonomic nervous system (ANS) is that part of the nervous system concerned with the control of involuntary functioning—the secretion of glands, beating of the heart, some part of respiration. The ANS is further divided into two, according to functioning: the sympathetic nervous system and the parasympathetic nervous system. Sympathetic nerve fibres usually constrict blood vessels, raise the blood pressure, dilate the pupils of the eye, depress the activities of the gastrointestinal tract, and increase the heart rate—the series of reactions occurring if one meets a lion, the fight or flight reaction! Parasympathetic fibres usually dilate the blood vessels, produce a fall in blood pressure, contract the pupils, increase gastrointestinal activity and slow the heart rate—the reaction of fainting; the direct opposite of sympathetic action.

Oesophagus A muscular tube passing from the back of the mouth to the stomach, carrying swallowed food and liquid.

Osteoarthritis See *Arthritis*.

Oxygen Normal constituent of air essential for respiration. See *Respiration*.

Pancreas Gland situated behind the stomach, producing two secretions, an external one—pancreatic juice which passes into the gut to assist digestion—and an internal one (in the islets of Langerhans) passing directly into the blood stream—insulin, which is essential for the metabolism of sugar and starches. Lack of insulin results in diabetes.

Paralysis Temporary or permanent loss of function. Voluntary movement depends upon normal functioning, i.e. on the impulse travelling from nerve cell in the brain along nerve fibre to muscle, with a relay station in the spinal cord. This pathway must be intact for a muscle to be under voluntary control. If a lesion occurs at the spinal cord level (relay station) the resultant paralysis is flaccid (with limp wasted muscles)—there is no tone in the muscle; if a lesion is at the brain level, the paralysis is spastic, i.e. stiff, with no wasting except what comes from disuse.

Parkinson's Disease A progressive disease of the central nervous system occurring in later life, in which the person becomes characteristically rigid. There is weakness, tremor, and very slow voluntary muscle reaction, but not real paralysis—though the effect is much the same.

Parathyroid Glands Four small glands situated at the back and on the lower edges of the thyroid gland in the neck. Their secretion regulates the metabolism of two elements in the blood: calcium and phosphorus. Where there is over-secretion, calcium is removed from the bones resulting in increased fragility.

Pelvis A bony basin consisting of the sacrum, the coccyx or tail, and the hip bones, which start on either side of the sacrum at the back and meet each other in the front. The basin contains the uterus (womb) and bladder and supports the spine, the lowest lumbar vertebra forming a joint with the sacrum. The hip bones form a ball and socket joint with the upper end of the thigh bone.

Perianal Muscles See *Anus*.

Peristalsis A progressive movement like a series of waves passing along the gut. The circular muscle in the gut wall 'behind' the wave contracts, while that 'in front of' the wave relaxes, and the contents of the gut—digested and undigested food in the small intestine, faeces in the large intestine—are forced onwards.

Plantar Appertaining to the sole of the foot—the plantar surface.

Plexus A network of nerves. See *Solar plexus*.

Premenstrual Tension Symptoms of varying degrees of intensity, all or some of which occur some days before menstruation starts—irritability, emotional tension, anxiety, depression, mood swings, swelling and soreness of the breasts, excessive appetite, head-ache. They subside when menstruation proper starts.

Psoas-iliacus muscle The powerful muscles which flex the thigh on to the abdomen. The psoas arises from the last thoracic and all the lumbar vertebrae, and is attached to a bony knob on the inside at the top of the thigh bone, while the iliacus arises from the inner edge of the hip bone and is attached like the psoas.

Psychotic Affected by a psychosis, that is a mental disorder of suffi-cient severity to result in some disintegration of the personality, or lack of contact with reality. Psychotics are therefore people who react antisocially or peculiarly in normal circumstances.

Rectum The lowest part of the large intestine. The rectum carries the faeces (food residue, bacteria, intestinal debris, mucus) from the rest of the large intestine to the anus, where it passes outside the body.

Renal System The body system concerned with excreting water and soluble waste products, comprising the two kidneys, the ureters taking urine from kidney to bladder, the bladder itself and the urethra leading from the bladder to the external opening through which the body gets rid of the urine. The urethra, nine inches long in the male, where it opens at the tip of the penis, is two inches long in the female where is opens at the front end of the vagina.

Respiration May be alveolar—external respiration—, or cellular—internal respiration. The former is the gaseous interchange wherein oxygen is taken from the air and replaced by carbon dioxide. In the lungs, across the walls of minute air spaces, or alveoli, the air comes into contact with the blood in which the red blood cells are carrying carbon dioxide—a waste product of metabolism in the body. The cells take the oxygen from the air, giving up the carbon dioxide. They then carry the oxygen round the body (see *Circulation of the blood*) and in the tissues give up the oxygen and take up carbon dioxide. This is cellular or internal respiration.

Respiratory System The body system whereby the gaseous inter-change of oxygen for carbon dioxide takes place, comprising mouth and nose, trachea (taking air down towards the lungs) which divides into right and left bronchus, just behind the top of the breastbone. Each bronchus subdivides into bronchi, smaller bronchi, bronchioles, and ultimately into minute air spaces called alveoli. Across the alveolar wall the red blood cells in the capillary blood vessels give up their waste carbon dioxide and take up oxygen, which they carry round to all the organs of the body, there giving up the oxygen for use and receiving the carbon dioxide—waste product of metabolism.

Retina A structure at the back of the eye sensitive to light. Light rays come to focus on the retina, having passed through the pupil. The brain interprets the images formed on the retina.

Rheumatoid Arthritis See *Arthritis*.

Rotation Turning on an axis. A limb can rotate either internally or externally on the axis of its point of contact with another bone, e.g. the hip joint.

Sacroiliac joints The joint between the sacrum and the hip bones on either side. A joint of very limited movement, easily disturbed, producing low back ache.

Solar Plexus A plexus (network) of nerves found behind the stomach, between the two suprarenal glands. It consists of two large ganglia from which sympathetic nerve fibres pass to the viscera (organs) in the abdomen.

Spastic A form of paralysis, where the lesion is higher than the relay station in the spinal cord; the paralysis is stiff not flaccid.

A term used loosely to denote a person with a disability due to brain damage, usually at birth, resulting in a greater or lesser degree of spastic paralysis.

Spina Bifida Congenital defect in the wall of the spinal canal, caused by failure of the sides of the vertebrae to close while the embryo is developing. As a result, at birth the spinal cord is exposed at the lower end of the back.

Spinal canal Spinal cord. See *Vertebra*.

Sternum A narrow flat bone in the middle of the front of the chest to which the ribs are joined by cartilage. Together with the ribs, their cartilages and the vertebrae from which the ribs arise, it forms the thoracic cavity, having the diaphragm below and the neck above.

Sternal notch A dip at the upper end of the breast bone.

Stroke Loss of consciousness followed by paralysis. It results from the rupture of an artery in the brain, or the formation of a clot within an artery in the brain. The degree of paralysis and the length of unconsciousness depend upon the size and site of the affected vessel.

Suprarenals (syn. adrenals) Triangular-shaped endocrine glands situated towards the midline, just above the kidneys. The gland has two parts, a medulla and a cortex. The medulla secretes adrenalin, the pouring of which into the blood produces the fight-flight reaction. It functions in conjunction with the sympathetic nervous system. The cortex has several secretions, among them cortisone, and has a profound effect upon all the body systems.

Systematic Disease A disease affecting the whole organism, the whole person, as opposed to a localised disease—like osteoarthritis affecting one joint only. Rheumatoid arthritis is systematic, affecting the body throughout, though it may manifest itself chiefly in the joints.

Tendon Strong fibrous tissue attaching muscles to bones,—the sinews. One of the strongest is the Achilles tendon attaching the calf muscles to the bone forming the heel.

Thorax That part of the body between the lower end of the neck and the diaphragm. The thoracic cavity is enclosed by the sternum, the rib cartilages and the ribs, the intercostal muscles and the twelve thoracic vertebrae.

Thyroid gland Endocrine gland situated in the neck above the larynx. Its secretion—thyroxin—regulates body metabolism.

Torso The trunk of the body, as distinct from the limbs and head.

Trachea The tube for the passage of air, running from the lower end of the larynx (voice box) to a point level with the fifth thoracic vertebra, where it divides into right and left bronchus, passing into right and left lungs respectively.

Trapezius Strong muscle of the upper spine, originating from the skull, the seventh cervical and all the thoracic vertabrae, and inserted into the collar bone and the shoulder blade. Its action is to draw the head backwards and to one or other side.

Umbilicus (syn. navel) A depression in the middle of the abdomen this is really a scar marking the point of attachment of the umbilical cord to the foetus, when in utero (womb).

Ureter A tube on either side of the body carrying urine from the kidney to the bladder. See *Renal system*.

Urethra A tube running from the bladder down the penis in the male, and down to the urethral opening in the female, for the excretion of urine. See *Renal system*.

Valve A membranous structure in the heart, capable of opening and closing, allowing the passage of blood in one direction only. There is a valve between the upper and lower chambers on each side of the heart, and one between the heart and the large arteries—the aorta, which discharges blood around the body from the left side of the heart—and the pulmonary arteries sending blood to the lungs from the right side of the heart. See *Circulation of the blood*.

Vertebra (pl. vertebrae) One of the 33 bones of the spinal column—seven cervical, 12 thoracic, five lumbar, five fused to form the sacrum, and four in the coccyx (rudimentary tail). Each vertebra has a body and an arch, and articulates with the vertebra above and the one below. There is an intervertebral disc between each vertebra and the next. The spinal cord, consisting of nerve cells and fibres, runs down the middle of the tube formed by the vertebra—the spinal canal; the spinal nerves pass out between the vertebrae.

Viscera Internal organs enclosed within a cavity e.g. abdominal viscera (liver, stomach) in the abdominal cavity, thoracic viscera (heart and lungs) in the thoracic cavity.

Appendix III

Sanskrit names for Yoga Postures

Many of the postures described in Chapter Five, Six and Seven have no Sanskrit names, as they are extracted from more complicated postures, or are just the beginnings of postures, or at the most half postures. The following, as described, are sufficiently near to the traditional posture for the name to be applicable. The word *asana*, which forms the second half of each name, means 'posture', the word *ardha*, which may precede it, means 'half', and the word *supta*, which also may precede it, means 'lying down'.

Archer	*Akarna Dhanurasana. Karna* means 'ear', *a* means 'to', and *dhanu* means 'bow'. In the posture the foot is pulled back like a bow string.
Back Stretch	*Paschimottanasana. Paschima* means 'the west', and refers to the back of the whole body (the eastern aspect of the body is the front). *Tan* means 'stretch' or 'extension'. Hence in the posture the back of the whole body, feet to crown, is stretched.
Beam	*Parighasana. Parigha* means a 'beam', or the bar used for shutting a gate.
Boat	*Ardha Navasana.* (The posture as described in Chapter Seven is really the half boat posture.) The word *Nava* means 'boat'.
Camel	*Ustrasana.* The word *ustra* means 'camel'.
Chest Stretch	*Parsvottanasana. Parsva* means 'side', *tan* means 'stretch' and *ut* means 'intense', 'extreme'—hence a posture which stretches the chest intensely.
Cobbler	*Baddha Konasana. Baddha* means 'caught', and *kona* means an 'angle'— the feet being caught by the hands and drawn in towards the perineum, the angle being the knee flexion presumably. The English name is very apposite as the position is used by Indian cobblers.

Cobra	*Bhujangasana* — this literally means 'serpent', and refers to the rearing up of a cobra before striking.
Cow's Head	*Gomukhasana. Go* means 'cow', *mukha* means 'face'. The name therefore means more the face of a cow rather than head of cow.
Dancer	*Natarajasana.* The word *nata* means a 'dancer', and *raja* means 'lord' or 'king'. Nataraja is the name given to Siva, the lord of the dance.
Dog	*Svanasana. Svana* is the word for 'dog'. A more complicated name is *Adha Mukha Svanasana*, where *Adha mukha* means 'having the face downwards'. In the posture the dog is stretching with the head and forelegs down, and the hind legs up!
Erect Posture	*Tadasana. Tada* means 'mountain', a pose where one stands as firm as a mountain. This is one of the two poses for which everybody seems to know the Sanskrit name.
Fish	*Matsyasana. Matsya* is the word for 'fish', and the pose is dedicated to Matsya the fish, an incarnation of Visnu, the source of the universe.
Floor Pose	*Savasana. Sava* means 'corpse'; actually the posture is full of latent vitality, and a great refresher of the organism. The word 'corpse' has been deliberately avoided throughout. Actually, this is the second posture of which everybody seems to know the Sanskrit name.
Half Moon	*Ardha Chandrasana. Ardha* means 'half', *Chandra* is 'the moon' — the curve in the posture does rather resemble a sickle moon. The posture does not really resemble an easier version of the Moon pose.
Hero	*Virasana. Vira* means 'warrior' or 'hero'.
Reclining Hero	*Supta Virasana. Supta* is a word for 'lying down'.
Lion	*Simhasana. Simha*, means 'lion'. This is a posture dedicated to the incarnation of Visnu as Man-Lion.
Locust	*Salabhasana. Salabha* is the word for 'locust'. In the pose a locust rests on the ground, tail in air.
Moon	*Chandrasana. Chandra* is 'the moon'. Strictly speaking the Sanskrit phrase *Ardha Chandrasana* is used for the Moon posture as described in this book, and not for the Half Moon as described.
Platform	*Purvottanasana. Purva* is the word for 'east' — the

front of the body from head to foot meaning east, as *Paschima* does 'the west'. *Ultana* means 'intense stretch'—as in Chest Stretch. Consequently the name means an intense stretch of the east side of the body—i.e. the front.

Shoulder Stand *Sarvangasana; Ardha Sarvangasana* being the half shoulder stand. Actually the complete title is *Salamba Sarvangasana*, where *alamba* means 'support', *sa* means 'with', *sarva* means 'whole' and *anga* means 'body'—i.e. the whole body propped up! It is in fact being propped on head, neck and shoulders only, with the hands as a support.

Spinal Twist *Marichyasama.* This is a posture dedicated to the wise man Marichi, son of Brahma the creator. The other Sanskrit words used for twists—*Matsyendrasana* and *Ardha Matsyendrasana*—denote a series altogether too strenuous and complicated for this book.

Squat *Utkatasana. Utkata* is a word meaning 'strong', and this fairly strenuous posture is meant to resemble sitting in a chair that isn't there. As described in the text, the trunk goes down lower than this to a complete squat—where possible.

Standing back stretch *Padangusthasana. Pada* means 'foot', and *angustha* is the 'big toe'. An early stage in the standing back stretch as described in the text is to hold on to the big toes.

Straight legs to floor *Jathara Parivartanasana. Jathara* means 'stomach', and *parivartana* means 'rolling round'. The posture is so named because the legs roll as it were round the belly, which is pulled over in the opposite direction.

Tree *Vrksasana. Vksa* is the word for 'tree'.

Triangle *Trikonasana. Tri* is 'three' and *kona* 'angle', three-angled meaning triangle. In actual fact, as described in the text the pose is *uttihita trikonasana*—the extended, stretched triangle.

Reverse Triangle *Pavritta Trikonasana.* The word *pavritta* means 'turned round'—which is exactly what the posture is, a turned round triangle pose.

Bibliography

Useful books — just a very few of the many hundreds to be found on the subject.

Light on Yoga, B. K. S. Iyengar, George Allen & Unwin
Pranayama, André van Lysebeth, Unwin Paperbacks
    (These two are a must for any teacher).
Teaching Yoga, Donald G. Butler, Pelham Books
The Authentic Yoga, P. Y. Deshpande, Rider and Company
Integral Yoga, Haridas Chaudhuri, George Allen & Unwin
    (Three interesting and helpful books well worth getting if you are building up a library on the subject).

For the student himself in the early stages, or the relatives of a handicapped student:

Key Facts Colour Guide (Yoga), Howard Kent, Cassell
Introduction to Yoga, Richard Hittleman, Bantam Books, pub. by arrangement with Workman Publishing Co. Inc.
Yoga for Health, Richard Hittleman, Hamlyn Publishing Group
Yoga in Ten Lessons, Déchamet, Search Press
Christian Yoga, Déchamet, Search Press
Yoga over Forty, Volin and Phelan, Sphere Books
Yoga and Health, Yesudian and Haitch, Unwin Paperbacks
Yoga Self Taught, André van Lysebeth, George Allen & Unwin
Yoga Some Basic Principles, Rawlinson, Combined Yoga Publications.
A Three Stage Course in Yoga, Malcolm Strutt, Centre for Conscious Living, Chippenham, Wilts
Yoga, Ernest Wood, Penguin Books
See and Be (Yoga for Children), Rachel Carr, Spectrum Books

None of these is difficult. Apart from the last, which deals with children, they are listed here starting with the very simplest and progressing — but not to anything abstruse. All are very readable, interesting and easily obtainable. It is simply a question of picking and choosing to suit yourself.

Index